Dr. Blaylock's

PRESCRIPTIONS

for Natural Health

Dr. Blaylock's
PRESCRIPTIONS
for
Natural Health

Russell L. Blaylock, MD

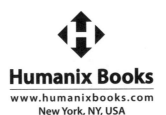

Humanix Books
www.humanixbooks.com
New York, NY, USA

Humanix Books

Dr. Blaylock's Prescriptions for Natural Heath
Copyright © 2016 by Humanix Books
All rights reserved

Humanix Books, P.O. Box 20989, West Palm Beach, FL 33416, USA
www.humanixbooks.com | info@humanixbooks.com

Library of Congress Cataloging-in-Publication Data

Blaylock, Russell L., 1945–
Dr. Blaylock's natural cures / Russell Blaylock.
   pages cm
 ISBN 978-1-63006-024-4 (tradepaper)
 1. Naturopathy--Popular works. 2. Alternative medicine--Popular works. 3. Self-
 care, Health--Popular works. I. Title. II. Title: Natural cures.
RZ440.B563 2015
615.5'35--dc23
                        2015026540

Interior design: Ben Davis

Humanix Books is a division of Humanix Publishing, LLC. Its trademark, consisting of the word "Humanix" is registered in the Patent and Trademark Office and in other countries.

Disclaimer: The information presented in this book is meant to be used for general resource purposes only; it is not intended as specific medical advice for any individual and should not substitute medical advice from a healthcare professional. If you have (or think you may have) a medical problem, speak to your doctor or healthcare practitioner immediately about your risk and possible treatments. Do not engage in any therapy or treatment without consulting a medical professional.

ISBN: 978-1-63006-024-4 (Paperback)
ISBN: 978-1-63006-025-1 (E-book)

Printed in the United States of America

Contents

Introduction

How to Use This Book

Natural cures have two equally important aspects: specific remedies for what ails you and a diet and lifestyle that enable your body to function well. A health condition, whether temporary or chronic, is a sign that things aren't working the way they're supposed to, and that changes need to be made. This book is designed to help you address both points, relieve symptoms, and identify and correct underlying diet and lifestyle habits that contribute to the problem and can perpetuate it.

Part I: Cornerstones of Health

This section has five chapters. I recommend you read these in full, no matter what type of situation you are seeking to resolve. It covers the most important, underlying elements that put an individual on a course toward health or disease. If you're suffering from a chronic condition, it's critical to do what you can to improve the situation. And, if you're in pretty good shape, the principles in these chapters will help you stay that way.

The power of nutrition is easy to underestimate. I've had many patients who adopted the principles I outline in chapters 1 through 3 and, just two weeks later, were amazed that they felt even better than they did in their youth.

Chapter 4 covers another very important aspect of nutrition: your doctor and media reports, both of which can make you doubt the value of dietary supplements. It explains why your doctor may be wary, why some media reports are negative, and how they don't paint an accurate picture. Chapter 5 describes hyperbaric oxygen treatment, which may help many conditions.

Part II: Natural Remedies for What Ails You

This makes up most of the book, and is organized by ailment. Here, you can simply look up the condition that concerns you or those you care about, and use the information to improve or prevent that condition. You will often see references to the first three chapters, in case you haven't read them.

The natural supplements in each section are designed to improve a specific condition. By themselves, they can bring about improvement, but taking them along with my recommended diet and lifestyle will deliver much more benefit. As an example, if you get headaches and are routinely eating a harmful food additive that is triggering the headaches, such as MSG, it makes sense to stop eating it. Otherwise, it's like trying to get pain relief while sitting on a sharp nail.

How Many Supplements Should You Take?

In this book and in my newsletter, I generally recommend numerous supplements for a given condition, and my readers often ask if they should take all of them. The answer is, no. It is best to start with one or maybe two and see if your condition will quickly clear. If so, all is well. For more resistant cases, simply add another of the recommended supplements and see if the combination will improve your results. And, never underestimate the power of healthy food.

PART 1

Cornerstones of Health

CHAPTER 1

The Anti-Aging Prescription

THE WESTERN DIET, HIGH in sugar, high-starch carbo-hydrates, inflammatory fats, and unhealthy red meats, is a prescription for chronic inflammation. This underlies every conceivable ill, from mild lack of energy and an inability to lose excess weight to heart disease, diabetes, arthritis, a compro-mised immune system, and every neurological condition. In short, it accelerates the aging process. Switching to an anti-in-flammatory diet reverses the process.

On a very basic level, the Western diet interferes with cellular energy production and fills the body with high levels of free radi-cals, highly reactive molecules that cause a process much like inter-nal rusting. Inflammatory substances and free radicals damage the major energy-producing components of cells, called mitochondria.

The best anti-inflammatory diet would include at least six serv-ings of vegetables, minimal sugar, only low-starch carbohydrates (starches), limited amounts of healthy meats and fish, and legumes. Purified water and white or green teas are good beverages, but you should avoid fruit juices, as they are high in sugar, fluoride, and, in many cases, aluminum. Moderate exercise should also be part of one's routine.

Below is an overview of the anti-inflammatory diet, which is also anti-aging. It includes exercise and some lifestyle issues, because these are part and parcel for controlling chronic inflammation, staying healthy, and slowing aging. In addition, the next two chapters cover two other vital aspects: excitotoxins, extremely harmful substances found mostly in food additives, and my favorite, easy way to add many more vegetables to your diet, with a vegetable drink. I've divided this information into three sections to make it easier to use.

Key Elements of an Anti-Inflammatory Diet

Eat and drink vegetables. Eat at least six servings of vegetables a day. These portions should include nutrient-dense ones, such as broccoli, Brussels sprouts, cauliflower, cabbage, onions, leeks, green lettuces, whole tomatoes, collards, mustard greens, spinach, kale, and celery. In addition, I recommend getting additional vegetables by using my vegetable drink recipe in chapter 3. Unlike juicing, it includes the natural fiber in vegetables, enables better absorption of nutrients, and makes it easy to increase your vegetable intake.

Eat the right meats. Saturated fats have very little connection to atherosclerosis or cholesterol, despite what your doctor may tell you. However, fats from organically raised meats are much safer than conventionally raised meats, as the latter have high levels of pesticides, herbicides, industrial chemicals, and toxic metals, and lower beneficial fats. The best diet would include limited amounts of organic chicken, turkey, fish, and some pork, no more than 6 ounces per day. Grass-fed beef could also be included about once a week. Lean cuts of meat are best.

I consider fish in the same category of foods as meat and recommend eating varieties that are low in mercury and high in anti-inflammatory omega-3 fats. Wild salmon is a good choice on both counts. Mercury levels in different fish change over time. The non-profit Environmental Working Group offers an updated seafood guide at www.ewg.org.

Know your fats. Unhealthy, inflammatory fats are omega-6 oils, used as cooking oils, in salad dressings, and in most processed foods. They include corn, safflower, sunflower, peanut, soybean, and canola oils, and be avoided. These oils oxidize very easily, meaning they degrade, much like margarine will turn rancid if you leave it out of the refrigerator. They are highly inflammatory within blood vessels, as well as the entire body. Check labels carefully, as many processed foods use an assortment of these oils.

Some omega-6 fats are essential, but most Western diets contain up to fifty times the amount needed. Vegetables and organically raised meats will supply all the omega-6 fats you need in a much healthier form than the ones in processed foods.

The best cooking oil is extra virgin coconut oil. If you do not like the taste of coconut, use refined coconut oil, which has no odor or taste. For salad dressings, use extra virgin olive oil.

Drink for health. Purified water and white or green teas are the best beverages. Water hydrates and cleanses without any liabilities. White and green teas contain antioxidants and anti-inflammatory substances that are therapeutic, as well as hydrating. If you are sensitive to caffeine or find that it keeps you up at night, choose decaffeinated versions. I don't recommend fruit juices, as they are high in sugar, fluoride, and, in many cases, aluminum.

Avoid trans fats. Listed as "partially hydrogenated" oils, these can be in many processed foods, even if a label claims zero trans fats. That's because food regulations allow a "zero" label if the amount of trans fat is less than 0.5 grams per serving. However, only a few grams of these per day can harm arteries, so eating several servings of foods that contain nearly one-half gram per serving can quickly add up to dangerous amounts. The best way to tell if the food really contains trans fat is to see if any partially hydrogenated oil is listed as an ingredient.

Avoid sugar. The strongest link to heart attacks, strokes, and atherosclerosis is not cholesterol or even fats, but sugar intake. Eliminate all sugar products, including cakes, pies, candy, sweetened drinks, fruit juices, and other sources. High fructose corn syrup should be avoided at all cost, as it is the worst culprit. Read ingredient labels carefully, as this form of sugar is not only in obviously sweet foods but also in many sauces, soups, and other foods we don't normally associate with sugar. Fruits are high in sugar and should be consumed only in limited amounts.

Minimize starchy carbohydrates. In the human body, some starches have the same effect as sugar. Foods high in starch are technically called "high-glycemic" carbohydrates, meaning they very rapidly convert to blood sugar after being eaten. These include breads (white or whole grain), buns, biscuits, rolls, crackers, chips, cereals, white rice, and potatoes.

Avoid fluoride. This includes fluorinated water, toothpaste, mouthwash, and black tea. Fluoride is a very reactive compound and even in very small concentrations can damage cells, tissues, and organs. This is especially true in children.

Maintain healthy teeth. Have regular dental checkups, routine cleanings, and take care of your teeth daily. This includes brushing after each meal and regular flossing. Chronic gum infections are strongly linked to chronic inflammation, atherosclerosis, heart attacks, and strokes.

Exercise regularly. Moderate exercise is best and should include resistance exercises that work all muscle groups. About 30 to 45 minutes of exercise on most days is beneficial. Extreme forms of exercise, such as extensive jogging, marathons, and triathlons, are not healthy and can actually make things worse, as they generate very high levels of damaging free radicals, which can persist for hours after the exercise.

Avoid prolonged, excessive stress. This is easier said than done in this crazy world. I recommend getting at least seven hours of sleep each night, praying regularly, and thinking about the beauty of the world. Soothing music is also a great stress reliever.

Stress causes an imbalance in the autonomic nervous system, which continually regulates all our organs, and puts our "fight or flight" response into overdrive. Chronic stress or acute intense stress generates high concentrations of free radicals. This leads to many of the problems associated with stress, such as ulcers, heart failure, arrhythmias, panic attacks, anxiety, depression, degeneration of the brain, and hypertension.

Everyday Natural Supplements

Throughout this book, I recommend various supplements for different health conditions. Theoretically, one can get adequate amounts of nutrients from food, especially with the addition of my vegetable drink recipe in chapter 3. However, if your diet falls short, as most do, these are some basic supplements for overall health. Unless you're trying to treat specific symptoms, which are covered in other sections of this book, I suggest following the usage directions for each product.

MULTIVITAMINS AND MINERALS

Chronic inflammation depletes many vitamins and minerals, yet these are needed to control and reduce inflammation. If you are eating 10 servings of nutrient-dense vegetables a day, a multivitamin and a mineral supplement can be overlooked. A multivitamin should include mixed carotenoids and a variety of B-vitamins, such as Extend Core, made by Vitamin Research Products.

FISH OIL

The most concentrated source of anti-inflammatory omega-3 fats, fish oil, helps to counteract the excess of pro-inflammatory fats and sugars in the Western diet. Although it isn't a substitute for avoiding inflammatory foods, it is an easy way to quell inflammation. If you suffer from an inflammatory condition or don't routinely eat wild salmon or other fish high in omega-3 fats a few times a week, a fish oil supplement is a good idea. One good product is liquid Norwegian fish oil, which comes in lemon and orange natural flavors, made by Carlson.

EXTRA VITAMIN C

Although multivitamins contain some vitamin C, extra amounts help to keep the immune system healthy and more resistant to viral and bacterial infections, and illness in general. One product that is well absorbed and easy on the stomach is Lypo-Spheric Vitamin C, made by LivOn Labs. It contains 1,000 mg of vitamin C in one single-serve packet of a gel, which can be mixed with water or juice. When taken in high doses, vitamin C should always be taken between meals, as it increases iron absorption when taken with food and can lead to iron overload.

VITAMIN D3

Vitamin D deficiency is quite widespread, yet this vitamin is vital for good health. Vitamin D plays an essential role in all tissues and organs of the body, including bones, the brain, the heart, and in immune function and protecting against cancer. In supplements, vitamin D3 is the form your body can absorb well and utilize. Before taking it as a supplement, I recommend getting your blood vitamin D level tested. This is a common test. The optimum level is between 65 ng/ml and 95 ng/ml. The dose of vitamin D3 needed depends on the degree of deficiency.

If the level is less than 30 ng/ml, the dose is 10,000 IU of vitamin D3 a day, taken with a meal, for three weeks, and then repeat the blood test. Once blood levels are in the target range, reduce the daily dose to 5,000 IU.

If the blood level is between 35 and 50 ng/ml, I recommend taking 5,000 IU a day for three to four weeks and then repeating the blood test. If levels are within the optimum range, reduce the dose to 2,000 IU a day.

MAGNESIUM

Magnesium is involved in more than 300 biochemical reactions in our bodies, yet it is widely lacking in our diets. It reduces inflammation, raises levels of our major internal antioxidant, glutathione, helps to keep arteries flexible, improves blood flow, and helps to prevent cramping and insomnia. The malate and citrate forms are more absorbable than others. A slow-release form such as Magnesium w/SRT, made by Jigsaw Health, is best for maintaining healthy magnesium levels in the body. Magnesium L-threonate has been shown to be the best form of the mineral for increasing brain levels. The two best sources are Neuro-Mag from Life Extension and Magnesium L-Threonate by Dr. Mercola.

There is another key issue that is ignored but critical to good health and plays a part in a great many conditions addressed in the rest of this book: excitotoxins. And that's the subject of the next chapter.

CHAPTER 2

Excitotoxins

FEW PEOPLE ARE AWARE of excitotoxins, yet these play a significant role in many of today's diseases. Excitotoxins are chemical substances that overstimulate certain types of cells in the brain, all of the nervous system, and many other organs, to such a degree that such cells become damaged or die. Dangerous amounts of these substances are found in common food additives, such as MSG, the artificial sweetener aspartame, and others.

The mechanism of excitotoxicity underlies many neurological conditions, such as Alzheimer's, Parkinson's, multiple sclerosis, strokes, brain trauma, autism, Gulf War syndrome, and Huntington's disease, and plays a critical role in many others, including migraines, diabetes, atherosclerosis, sudden death from heart disease, eye diseases, digestive disorders, autoimmune disorders, growth of tumors, spread of cancer, and obesity.

MSG was first found to be an excitotoxin in 1957, when two eye doctors discovered that it destroyed the inner nerve layer of the retina in mice, especially in young animals. At the time, MSG was routinely added to baby food, as well as being broadly used in adult foods. As a result of the research, food manufacturers began to withdraw MSG from baby food, but it has continued to be widely used in other packaged and processed foods to enhance taste.

In 1969, research by Dr. John Olney showed that when newborn mice were exposed to MSG, they did not develop normally, but were very short and obese, and suffered brain damage. Since then, many other studies have found that MSG and other excitotoxins play critical roles in disease.

The Most Common Excitotoxin: Glutamate

Glutamate is the key component of MSG that causes damage. However, glutamate is also a neurotransmitter, a chemical that is naturally produced in our bodies and transmits signals between brain and nerve cells and other cells. In fact, it is the most commonly used neurotransmitter in the brain.

How can such a natural substance cause problems? We need a certain amount of it to function normally, but too much causes cells to become overexcited, leading to damage and eventual cell death. An excess can come from two sources: overproduction in our bodies, as a result of an injury or disorder, and too much glutamate in our diet. Since this mechanism plays a major role in many health conditions, it is important to have some understanding of how it works.

Although most people are not familiar with excitotoxicity, it has become a widely studied area, with decades of research focusing mainly on the brain and nervous system. I have studied the subject for more than 25 years and have found that the mechanism can also affect every organ in the human body. To describe this process in many parts of the body, not just the brain and nervous system, I coined the term "immunoexcitotoxicity."

What Is Immunoexcitotoxicity?

This is a combination of two mechanisms: excitotoxicity and inflammation. You may be familiar with the idea that chronic inflammation lays the groundwork for many diseases, including heart disease, diabetes, and cancer, and plays a major role in chronic pain. When inflammation is combined with excitotoxicity, the effect is even more damaging, and this is what I named immunoexcitotoxicity.

In many conditions described in this book, I refer to glutamate, excitotoxins, excitotoxicity, and immunoexcitotoxicity. Each of these terms relates to the same mechanism, but in different ways. To avoid confusion, this is what each one means:

Glutamate: A chemical substance produced by our bodies and found in overabundant amounts in MSG and some other food additives and ingredients (see the list below).

Excitotoxin: A substance that causes cells to become overexcited to the point of becoming damaged or dead. Glutamate is a very prevalent excitotoxin. Others include aspartic acid in aspartame, an artificial, zero-calorie sweetener, L-cysteine, homocysteine, and other cysteine metabolic products.

Excitotoxicity: The process of cells becoming overexcited, to a point that is damaging or deadly.

Immunoexcitotoxicity: The combination of excitotoxicity and inflammation, which underlies and/or perpetuates many disease processes. Inflammation always triggers excitotoxicity in the nervous system.

These are some key areas where immunoexcitotoxicity occurs and damages health:

- In the lining of blood vessels, contributing to atherosclerosis

- In the lungs, contributing to respiratory problems

- In the pancreas, contributing to diabetes

- In endocrine glands, where it disrupts the function of hormones and appetite, contributing to obesity

- In the eyes, contributing to vision disorders, such as glaucoma, and vision loss

- In the brain and nervous system, contributing to neurological disorders such as Alzheimer's, Parkinson's, ALS, and multiple sclerosis

- In the digestive system, contributing to various digestive disorders, such as irritable bowel diseases

- In the immune system, contributing to autoimmune disorders, such as lupus

- In tumors, enhancing their growth and spread of cancer

How Diet Influences Excitotoxicity

The glutamate in MSG is the most prevalent excitotoxin in our diet, in processed and packaged foods. Yet, I have heard a number of people remark that they are not sensitive to MSG. Usually that means it doesn't cause them to have a headache or other symptoms of the "Chinese restaurant syndrome," at least not right after they consume the MSG. In fact, people who develop the Chinese restaurant syndrome are the lucky ones, because they know to avoid the food additive.

Studies show that for most people, it takes about an hour for the effects of one dose of MSG to manifest inside the human body, but one dose may not produce any noticeable symptoms. However, because many foods contain MSG, most Americans are continually exposed to excess amounts of the chemical, and it silently causes harm.

Let's say you eat several foods containing MSG, such as flavored potato or corn chips, a frozen dinner, and a commercial or canned soup. Your blood glutamate will rise, perhaps

20-fold. Careful studies have shown that when you combine foods containing MSG with aspartame, the ingredient in popular zero-calorie sweeteners in diet sodas, blood glutamate levels are double what they would be if you ingested MSG alone. So, if you add a diet drink, glutamate then increases to 40-fold or 4,000 percent! People do this all the time, especially young people.

Certain nutrients, especially magnesium and nutrients found in vegetables without pesticides, bolster the human body's ability to deal with MSG, but these tend to be lacking in the American diet, especially among people who favor processed and fast food. This enhances the negative, excitotoxic effect of MSG.

Who Is Most Susceptible?

Exposure to excitotoxins—MSG and aspartame being the most prevalent in our food supply—is always harmful, and the combination of these two ingredients doubles the damage. This means that a diet filled with excitotoxic food additives causes you to age much faster and more intensely than normal, and increases your risk of developing a chronic disease. However, there are two stages of life where human beings are most susceptible: during the early years and after age 50.

Many studies have shown that glutamate plays a major role in how the brain is formed during development, and babies and young children face lifelong damage from exposure to glutamate. Exposure can begin in the womb, where MSG and other excitotoxins consumed by the mother are transferred through the placenta, leading to abnormal learning, addiction risk, behavioral and emotional problems, endocrine problems, and much higher risk of obesity later in life.

After age 50, the body's ability to tolerate excitotoxins declines. This is also a time when levels of chronic inflammation are likely higher, and with excitotoxins in food, the combination accelerates development of disease.

Fortunately, exposure to excitotoxins can be dramatically reduced by avoiding the most common food additives that deliver excessive amounts of glutamate. If you routinely eat fast food, prepare meals with canned or packaged foods, or drink sodas, bottled iced teas, or other flavored beverages, it will require some effort to transform your diet. But it's a realistic approach. Once you become aware of what is in your staples and find additive-free versions, it will become routine.

Food Ingredients to Avoid

The use of excitotoxic additives is so widespread that there are only two ways to avoid them: by reading the list of ingredients on food labels and choosing additive-free products and by eating only freshly prepared foods. MSG, or monosodium glutamate, may be listed as such, but glutamate may be disguised under another name. These are some common ingredients that contain glutamate and should be avoided:

- Amino acid chelates (in some mineral supplements)
- Autolyzed yeast
- Brewer's yeast
- Broth
- Bullion
- Calcium caseinate
- Carrageenan
- Condensed milk
- Enzymes (listed as a food ingredient, not the same as digestive enzyme supplements)
- Hydrolyzed oat flour
- Hydrolyzed protein
- Hydrolyzed soy protein

- Hydrolyzed vegetable protein
- Malt extract
- Malted barley
- Malted milk
- Milk powder
- Mushroom powders
- Natural flavoring (only includes truly natural flavoring ingredients)
- Plant protein extract
- Seasoning made from powdered tomatoes
- Sodium caseinate
- Soy protein concentrate
- Soy protein isolate
- Soy sauce
- Stock
- Textured protein
- Tomato powder
- Whey protein concentrate, isolate, or extract
- Yeast extract

Many diet drinks and foods, or those labeled "reduced calorie" or "sugar free," are sweetened with aspartame, another excitotoxin which should be avoided. These include many sodas, iced teas, fruit drinks, jams, jellies, flavored yogurts, baked and frozen desserts, puddings, syrups and other toppings, and some seemingly healthy nutritional bars and drinks. In addition, MSG or glutamate may be (but are not always) in ingredients listed as "seasoning" or "spices."

Some meat products, including whole chicken and turkey and some beef products, are soaked, painted, or injected with

MSG-containing substances. In addition, portobello mushrooms are naturally high in glutamate—the harmful component of MSG.

Buying organic foods is a simple way to avoid excitotoxic additives, but it isn't always possible. As a rule of thumb, fresh vegetables, grown without herbicides or pesticides, or peeled where possible, and always washed, are a safe bet. Organic or grass-fed meat and poultry are good options, but check the methods used by the supplier. For any food product, the label and a company's website are useful sources of information, and if in doubt, call the food producer and ask.

For more information and updates about sources of MSG, check out www.truthinlabeling.org.

Foods High in Glutamate

Many foods naturally contain significant amounts of glutamate that can make digestive disorders worse when eaten in excess, especially when the food is processed, fermented, or slow cooked. In general, raw whole foods, even though they may contain significant levels of glutamate, are safe because the glutamate is released slowly, thus preventing an overload of glutamate in the blood stream. Liquid forms of glutamate, such as soy sauce and aspartame-sweetened sodas, are rapidly absorbed and more harmful.

Here are some foods that are naturally high in glutamate:

- All meats, but especially red meats

- Meat gravies and meat-based sauces

- All mushrooms, but especially portobello mushrooms

- All cheeses, but especially parmesan and gorgonzola cheeses

- Packaged sauces, especially white and tomato sauces

- Powdered and pureed tomatoes (whole tomatoes are generally safe)

- Many nuts, especially peanuts, cashews, and walnuts. These also contain many beneficial substances and minerals, and should be eaten only in moderation. Be warned that some brands of peanuts contain added MSG.

Many people don't experience problems when eating these foods in moderation. However, we each have a different tolerance level.

More Ways to Protect Yourself

Avoiding excitotoxic food additives is the first step. Because of the way excitotoxicity works, we know that people who have poor overall nutrition or are exposed to other toxins, such as pesticides, are much more affected by excitotoxic food additives. Eating a wholesome diet is part and parcel of protecting your health.

Organic foods, and those produced without pesticides or additives, are the best choices. Although these are not the majority of packaged foods on supermarket shelves and in popular chain restaurants, it pays to seek out additive-free versions. Increasing your intake of nutrient-packed vegetables is an essential way to give yourself additional protection. I've found that an easy way to do this is to make your own concentrated vegetable drink, covered in detail in the next chapter.

CHAPTER 3

Drink Your Veggies

A MASSIVE AMOUNT OF RESEARCH has been done on the health benefits of fruits and vegetables. What we have learned is that fruits, and especially vegetables, contain literally thousands of compounds that have important medicinal and health-giving value.

In the beginning, researchers searched for the one compound that would account for the beneficial effects, but now they have discovered that it is usually the combination of these components—such as vitamins, minerals, flavonoids, and other special molecular compounds—that provides the greatest benefits. Each nutrient plays a special role in protecting cells, tissues, and organs.

Isolated compounds can have some incredible effects, as you'll see with various supplements covered in later sections, but the core of your health program should be your diet.

Vegetables appear to be the most beneficial. I recommend maximizing your intake of these wonderful compounds. One of the more beneficial sources of nutrients and special health-giving molecules is berries, including blueberries, raspberries, blackberries, and muscadine berries, as these also have tremendous health benefits.

Most authorities suggest we eat at least 5 to 10 servings of fruits and vegetables a day and for those over age 65, 15 servings a day. Serving sizes differ, depending on the consistency of the vegetable:

- Loose vegetables, such as greens, serving size: 1 cup

- Dense vegetables, such as cauliflower, Brussels sprouts, and broccoli, serving size: ½ cup

Solving the Veggie Problem

As you can see, 10 or 15 daily servings of vegetables would constitute a very large volume, more than most people can eat. And, there is another problem: the nutrients in veggies are not easily absorbed.

The important nutrients in vegetables, and all plant foods, are located inside cells. Each cell is encased in a cell wall that people cannot digest. As a result, we normally absorb only about 10 percent of the nutrients when we eat raw vegetables. Cooking will break the cells open and release most of the nutrients, but many nutrients, such as the vitamins, are destroyed by the heat.

The best solution is to blenderize your vegetables and berries, meaning blend them with water until they turn into liquid. This way, all the nutrients are released into the solution and are not damaged by heat. Studies have shown that drinking blenderized vegetables increases absorption of the plant nutrients to as much as 80 percent. This means that you can drink a much smaller amount of the blenderized mix and still get all the nutrients you would normally get by eating 10 to 15 servings of vegetables and berries.

Why not Juice?

I am frequently asked why I don't recommend juicing. First, I think juicing is a good way to get a high concentration of nutrients, but I have a problem with the fact that you are throwing away a lot of useful plant fiber. The fiber is a powerful inhibitor of colon cancer and other diseases, such as diabetes. Second, juicing is a messy process. Blenderizing is a lot easier and the cleanup is much faster.

Always Wash Produce

In general I recommend that you only use organically grown produce, but even then, it is important to wash all vegetables and fruits, as they will have some pesticide and herbicide residues, just from the contaminants in the atmosphere. A commercial vegetable wash is fine. Non-organic vegetables require a more thorough washing. Some vegetables will have a wax coating which can be impregnated with pesticides and herbicides, and this can be scrubbed off with a vegetable brush.

Getting Started

For the beginner, until your body gets accustomed to blenderized vegetables, I recommend starting with a more diluted drink. Otherwise, the high fiber content and high concentration of vegetables can cause diarrhea. To prevent this, I suggest filling your blender with cold, distilled or filtered water to the halfway mark, and using only three vegetables plus a berry concentrate. The concentrate adds flavor as well as nutrients. The one I recommend below contains less sugar than whole blueberries or other blueberry concentrates—around 5 grams per tablespoon.

Beginner's Drink Recipe

This will be a watery solution, but it will allow your gut to adjust. For the first three days, drink 8 ounces, once daily, then drink 8 ounces, twice daily, for the rest of the week.

INGREDIENTS:

- Distilled or filtered water
- 4 stalks organic washed celery
- ½ head organic washed cauliflower
- 1 cup organic washed kale
- 4 ounces Fruit Fast blueberry concentrate from www.brownwoodacres.com

1. Fill the blender halfway with water.
2. Add celery, cauliflower, and kale.
3. Blend to mix well, for 1 minute. Do not leave the blender on longer as it will heat the water and damage some of the nutrients.
4. Add the blueberry concentrate and blend on a low speed for 1 minute.
5. Drink 8 ounces.

Keep leftover drink mix in the refrigerator and make more when you've run out. After the first week, progress to the full, thicker blend with more veggies.

How to Make the Full Blend

The Best Veggies list contains the most beneficial ones but you can add others for variety, according to your personal preferences. I generally blend at least six different vegetables and the blueberry concentrate. Always start by filling your blender with cold, distilled or filtered water to the halfway mark, then add veggies one at a time, and, finally, add the blueberry concentrate and blend on low for another minute.

How many vegetables you blend depends on your goals. If you have a serious inflammatory disorder or cancer, you will want to add more veggies, and a greater variety.

From the Best Veggies list, choose at least three of the vegetables. For things like celery, use at least 10 stalks. After filling the blender half-full with water, put celery stalks in the blender and blend until you have a liquid. Then add kale, at least four cups, and blend it to a liquid. Continue adding vegetables until you have a rather thick green blend. You can add more water as necessary to bring it to a consistency you can easily drink.

> **BEST VEGGIES**
>
> These are the top anti-cancer and brain-protecting vegetables. Start with three, and after a week, add two more. Vary them over time, according to your personal preferences.
>
> - Artichoke
> - Broccoli
> - Brussels sprouts
> - Cabbage
> - Cauliflower
> - Celery
> - Collard greens
> - Kale
> - Parsley
> - Spinach
> - Squash

For a smoother drink with a pleasant taste, add three squash and/or half a head of cabbage.

Once all the veggies are blended, add about 4 ounces of blueberry concentrate. Blueberries contain powerful antioxidants called anthocyanins, which reduce inflammation and protect a number of organs, especially the heart and brain.

SAVING YOUR VEGETABLE BLEND

I usually blend a fresh batch once a week and keep it in the fridge. However, when frozen, the drink will keep in the freezer for several weeks. I have had some patients who frequently traveled for work and needed a way to store the blenderized veggie drink. Also, if you do not want to make the drink fresh every day, you can store as much as you would like in your freezer for several weeks.

To freeze, divide the drink into Ball jars. Be sure to leave about one inch of space at the top of the jar to allow for expansion of the liquid as it freezes. Jars can be transferred to the refrigerator to thaw, as needed.

Drinking your vegetable blend each day is an easy way to get protective amounts of nutrients and fiber from whole, raw veggies. And, your body will absorb a lot more vitamins, minerals, and other wonderful compounds.

CHAPTER 4

The War on Alternative Medicine

IN THE MEDIA, WE often hear the terms "orthodox medicine" and "alternative medicine," as if they were mutually exclusive. Worse still is the impression, and sometimes the outright statement, that "alternative medicine" is non-scientific, and therefore not based on clinical or scientific evidence. Today's so-called orthodox medical practitioners coined the term "evidence-based medicine" to imply that only their practice is based on science, but this is not the case.

In fact, a great deal of alternative medicine is based on very well demonstrated scientific evidence, while much of orthodox medicine is based on fads and perpetuated myths. For example, most doctors, and especially oncologists, endlessly repeat the mantra that antioxidant supplements interfere with traditional cancer treatments even though there is, except for a few instances, no clear scientific evidence that this is true. In fact, the opposite is generally true.

We see this same mythology in statements about vitamin dangers, such as "vitamin D3 and vitamin A in moderately higher doses are dangerous." Examination of the scientific evidence shows that these statements are not true and never have been. Claims that vitamin C causes kidney stones have also been proven false. Studies quoted by orthodox doctors only refer to vitamin C in a test tube. In people, the vitamin does not cause kidney stones because we have different metabolic systems.

A clue to the weakness of any argument is when one side resorts to name-calling, double standards of proof, and in particular, the use of the courts and lawmakers to stifle opposing viewpoints. Being that most of the media, regulatory agencies, the courts, and politicians are on the side of so-called orthodox medicine, the battle is quite lopsided. What gets buried in this battle is the truth.

What We Have Learned about Natural Treatments

When I first became interested in alternative treatments more than 50 years ago, little scientific data existed to support the claims of practitioners of this medical art. Most of the literature was in the form of self-published books, pamphlets, and obscure lectures given in local settings. Most authors of these works were little-known PhDs, naturopaths, and herbalists, people with few recognized medical credentials—yet, subsequent studies have most often shown they were correct all along.

Things have been changing. Recently, a professor at a medical school told his students that most of these "alternative" treatments have been used for thousands of years, that few modern medicines have had such a long history of success, and that such clinical evidence should not be ignored. He was right on target.

Over the past 30 years, a great deal of research has been done on many of the extracts used in alternative medicine to see how they often produce dramatic effects on human disease. For example, hawthorn tea has been used successfully for centuries to treat "dropsy," an older term for heart failure. We now understand, on a molecular and cellular level, how it works this miracle.

Hundreds of such compounds have now been intensively studied. Not only are these plant extracts, vitamins, and minerals quite potent in fighting disease, but they are much safer than the pharmaceutical drugs making up the backbone of "orthodox medicine."

It has been estimated that more than 100,000 people die every year as a result of taking pharmaceutical drugs in the prescribed doses, and this number excludes allergic reactions. Only a handful of deaths or serious complications have been associated with natural products and most of these were due to taking abusive doses far in excess of what has been recommended.

How Natural Products Beat Drugs

Pharmaceutical drugs have very little, if any, ability to prevent disease, whereas many natural products have very powerful preventive properties. Most diseases can be prevented or their risk can be greatly reduced by consuming large amounts of nutrient-dense vegetables and some selected fruits. However, pharmaceutical drugs are designed to treat diseases once they have become full blown. Worse still, most drugs do not address the cause of the disease, but only treat symptoms.

I often hear alternative health proponents say that headaches are not caused by a lack of ibuprofen and heart failure is not caused by a lack of beta blockers. Nevertheless, the person with a headache is thankful that the medication provides relief, and the person with heart failure is grateful for the beneficial effects of beta-blockers. But many plant extracts also treat symptoms.

As an example, hawthorn contains chemicals that stimulate the heart muscle to contract with more effective force, just like certain heart drugs, but it also stimulates dilation of blood vessels to improve blood flow. And the herb does these things with very few adverse effects, whereas cardiac drugs can have a number of severe, often deadly, side effects. And unlike the cardiac drugs, hawthorn can also reduce inflammatory factors in the blood that actually cause heart failure, thereby correcting a major cause of the disease. Hawthorn's other "side effects" are mostly beneficial, such as protecting the brain, decreasing risk of cancer, and reducing harmful overreaction of the immune system.

We see this with a number of natural compounds. For example: curcumin is a brain protectant that also reduces inflammation in other areas of the body, has antibacterial and antiviral effects, reduces atherosclerosis, protects against radiation damage, improves cellular energy production, is a potent antioxidant, and is a powerful anti-cancer agent. Magnesium is critical for the operation of hundreds of enzymes in our bodies, is anti-inflammatory, increases levels of our internal antioxidants, reduces blood clots, opposes allergies, reduces autoimmune inflammation, stimulates cellular energy production, protects the heart muscle, reduces atherosclerosis, and protects the brain. No pharmaceutical drug can say the same. Most drug side effects are quite harmful and some are deadly.

Where Drugs Excel

Purists on both sides of this argument reject the use of any of their opponents' remedies. I think this is an error. Modern orthodox medicine excels in treating acute conditions—diseases and injuries that occur suddenly, such as a heart attack, trauma, emergency surgery, or an infection. A number of medicines can be life-saving, such as insulin for insulin-dependent diabetes or antibiotics for treating infections.

The greatest strides in medicine came with the introduction of antibiotics. Previously, the leading killer of Americans in the 1920s through the 1950s was infection. When I was growing up, a number of people in our community died of pneumonia, but if antibiotics had been available then, they likely would not have died.

Despite the healing power of antibiotics, alternative practitioners have learned that abuse of these drugs has now produced new problems which can be very serious. For example, the destruction of beneficial probiotic organisms in the colon can have devastating effects on health and can prevent the proper development of the immune system in babies. Vaccinations have now produced a great variety of medical disorders, from autoimmune diseases, diabetes, and leukemia to brain degeneration and possibly even autism spectrum disorders. We cannot afford to ignore these harmful effects.

Why Orthodox Medicine Isn't Enough

Alternative medicine can and should work along with orthodox medicine. The best way to demonstrate this is with an example of a situation that often arises.

Let's say Bill develops pneumonia. He is not a devotee of good diets and hates to exercise. In essence, he is the quintessential couch potato. He smokes a pack of cigarettes and drinks a few beers every day, and more on the weekends. His wife tries to get him to take a multivitamin every day but he adamantly refuses.

Bill is seen in the emergency room and immediately admitted. His sputum is cultured and he is given an antibiotic. For the first few days, he seems to be getting better, but then his condition worsens. Subsequent cultures show that he now has several harmful organisms growing in his lungs. Newer antibiotics are added and he is moved to the intensive care unit. No vitamins are added to his IV fluids and his appetite is poor. Of course, he is eating the most nutrient-deficient, tasteless food in the known universe—hospital food. The peas are like wax and the mashed potatoes taste like wallpaper paste.

His doctors are puzzled by why Bill continues to deteriorate, despite getting three powerful broad-spectrum antibiotics. After a month in the hospital and with an ever-expanding list of medications, Bill finally begins to turn the corner and eventually returns home to resume his self-destructive lifestyle.

Why Alternative Medicine Is Essential

What could have been different? Let's take it from the beginning. Most important, Bill could have changed his diet years ago to one that promoted health, especially immunity. However, Bill ate a lot of foods cooked in omega-6 oils, such as corn, safflower, sunflower, peanut, or soybean oil, which suppress the immunity needed to fight infections and that promote silent, chronic inflammation.

Bill could have gone easy on other ingredients on the bad-guy list: simple sugars, such as table sugar, and dextrose and high fructose corn syrup added to hundreds of commercial foods. High intake of sugar also suppresses immunity, feeds harmful bacteria, and can aggravate inflammation. (This is why diabetics have such a high incidence of infections and have difficulty recovering from them.)

Other commercial food additives, prevalent in Bill's unhealthy diet, can also lower resistance to infections and impair recovery. These include MSG (monosodium glutamate), fluoride (in water as well as some processed foods), sulfates and sulfites, food dyes, aluminum, cadmium, mercury, and lead. Fluoride, for example, impairs immune cell function, interferes with many aspects of normal cell function, worsens inflammation, and damages many tissues and organs, especially the heart and brain.

Excess numbers of vaccinations can also significantly impair immune function and increase the risk of developing an uncontrollable infection. Vaccinations can push the immune system beyond resistance, into a suppressed mode of operation.

By eating a wholesome diet of natural foods and avoiding substances that impair his own immunity, Bill's resistance to infection would have been higher, and perhaps he could have avoided pneumonia. At the very least, with the help of antibiotics, his body would have been better equipped to fight it off more rapidly, with less suffering.

It's Never Too Late

Once in the hospital with pneumonia, Bill can't turn back the clock on his unhealthy lifestyle, but his recovery could be considerably improved with alternative medicine. Remember, his infection didn't resolve easily.

Although antibiotics are essential in Bill's situation, natural immune stimulants can boost the ability of his body to fight harmful bacteria and have been shown to greatly improve recovery from major infections. Keep in mind that antibiotics do a great job in killing harmful bacteria (with the side effect of also killing beneficial ones), but they don't enhance the body's innate ability to resist or fight infection.

One effective immune stimulant is called beta-glucan (technically beta-1,3/1,6-glucan), which is most commonly derived from the cell wall of yeast. Others include larch tree extract, Carnivora (a special European plant extract, made by Carnivora Research International), IP-6 (inositol-6 phosphate, a vitamin-like component of plant fibers), and extracts from shitake and maitake mushrooms. They act quickly and produce sustained boosting of the immune system.

Infections and the related stress will severely and rapidly deplete essential nutrients, such as vitamin C, the B vitamins, and magnesium, which further reduces the body's ability to recover. Poor Bill was in a state of extreme vulnerability because of his diet and couch-potato lifestyle, so when the infection hit him, his defenses were severely impaired.

The Power of Supplements

You have to think of an infection as a war zone, where the bombs and bullets are flying in every direction and also harm innocent bystanders. All this carnage has to be cleaned up and damaged tissues must be repaired. This requires good hydration to help eliminate waste products and a lot of nutrients and minerals, which supplements can quickly provide.

High-dose vitamin C will quickly replace losses and plays a major role in fighting infections without triggering excessive, harmful immune reactions. I recommend Lypo-Spheric Vitamin C, made by LivOn Labs. The B vitamins can also be replaced rapidly, either by taking a high-dose multivitamin by mouth or having it added to IV fluids. These vitamins are water soluble and levels rise quickly.

The fat-soluble vitamins take a little longer to be replaced, but mixing them with extra virgin olive oil or coconut oil will greatly improve absorption. These include vitamin D3, vitamin E in the form of mixed tocopherols and tocotrienols, and vitamin A. Replacement of these essential vitamins not only improves tissue and organ defenses, but also reduces the damage done by the infection and by the immune system while it's fighting off harmful invaders.

Magnesium is essential for tissue and organ protection during an infection and can reduce excess inflammation. Studies have shown that when magnesium levels are low, we can't produce adequate levels of our chief internal antioxidant, called glutathione, and this further reduces the body's ability to recover.

NAC, short for N-acetyl-L-cysteine, is a nutrient that boosts our natural production of glutathione. Studies have shown that, by doing this, NAC can significantly shorten the length of an infectious illness, especially viral illnesses.

During and after an infection, it's vital to take large doses of probiotics, beneficial bacteria in the digestive system. These are killed off by antibiotics, which results in overgrowth of harmful bacteria and yeast, making an infection more difficult to control.

Using natural treatments, there are a great number of things one can do to reduce the chances of developing a serious infection, and should it happen, to treat it effectively. Combining alternative methods with orthodox treatments gives the best chance of an excellent outcome and a lower risk of recurrence.

CHAPTER 5

Hyperbaric Oxygen Therapy

HYPERBARIC OXYGEN THERAPY IS recommended for many conditions described in this book. Called HBOT for short, this is a medical treatment that uses pure oxygen under greater than normal atmospheric pressure. It is effective and safe for many different types of ailments. Lack of sufficient oxygen may damage tissues—in the brain when a stroke occurs, for example—and contribute to a variety of diseases, complications, or side effects of medical treatment. HBOT can help to heal and restore function, to varying degrees, and new applications for such treatment are continually being found.

HBOT is administered in hyperbaric chambers. These are medical devices with solid, hard walls that deliver 100 percent oxygen. The patient sits or lies in the chamber and breathes pure oxygen for a prescribed period of time. Depending on individual needs, patients may receive only one treatment or

many, during a span of days, weeks, or even months, at prescribed intervals. The atmospheric pressure in the chamber is
higher than normal. Some hyperbaric chambers are designed
to treat one patient and others can simultaneously treat several people.

There are also soft, inflatable chambers, sometimes sold for
home use, which contain only 21 percent oxygen—the same
amount of oxygen that is in the air we normally breathe. Such
soft chambers are not medical hyperbaric chambers and don't
deliver the same benefits.

How It Works

Oxygen has the power to heal, but damaged tissues can suffer
from a short supply, and normal breathing of our air (which is
only 21 percent oxygen) doesn't deliver sufficient amounts. The
principle of HBOT is this: in a hyperbaric chamber, the air pressure can be increased up to three times our normal air pressure.
This increased pressure enables pure oxygen to saturate red
blood cells and plasma, a colorless liquid that makes up part of
the blood and other fluids in our circulatory system. As a result,
oxygen is able to reach places that might otherwise be deprived
and inaccessible.

Studies have shown that hyperbaric oxygen has a number of
beneficial properties, such as reducing tissue swelling, reducing
inflammation, killing infectious organisms, strengthening connective tissue and bone, and promoting wound healing.

The FDA has approved HBOT treatments for many conditions, such as carbon monoxide poisoning, gas gangrene, crush
injuries, wound healing, resistant osteomyelitis, skin grafts,
burns, decompression sickness, and brain abscesses. Researchers and health practitioners have also found a number of other conditions that respond to HBOT, including autism, ALS,
ADHD, anxiety, bladder infections, and brain injuries. In general, HBOT can help with any malady that is associated with

decreased oxygenation, poor blood supply, infection, inflammation, or damage to the nervous system.

Where to Get HBOT

Hyperbaric oxygen treatment centers may be found in independent clinics, hospitals, and affiliated outpatient centers. Not all conditions are treated at every facility, so it is important to find an appropriate center with doctors and other personnel who are well trained and have significant experience in treating all aspects of a given condition. For example, physical therapy or other treatment may be required, along with HBOT, in stroke rehabilitation. In all cases, a hyperbaric chamber with hard walls is the essential medical device.

- For a list of centers treating FDA-approved conditions, visit www.hyperbariclink.com.

- For a list of centers treating a broader range of conditions, visit www.healing-arts.org/children/hyperbaricoxygen therapy_hbot.htm.

- To locate a center near you, call the International Hyperbarics Association at 877- IHA-USA1 (877-442-8721) or visit www.ihausa.org.

PART 2

Natural Remedies
for What Ails You

CHAPTER 6

Men's Health

» Prostate Disorders
» Erectile Dysfunction

Prostate Disorders

Men, especially as they age, are often affected by prostate problems, most often prostate enlargement, chronic prostatitis, or prostate-related pelvic pain. In all these conditions, studies have identified elevated levels of inflammatory chemicals in prostate tissue, indicating that chronic inflammation is a common denominator. Inflammation is also linked to prostate cancer. Drugs and natural substances that reduce inflammation also reduce prostate enlargement, prostatitis, and pelvic pain.

Almost all men experience some degree of prostate enlargement as they get older. The gland surrounds the urethra, the tube through which urine flows, and when enlarged, exerts pressure upon this tube, impairing the ability to urinate. Chief symptoms are difficulty emptying the bladder and more frequent trips to the bathroom, which can be annoying during the day and can disturb sleep at night.

Benign prostatic hyperplasia—BPH for short—is another name for the condition. With BPH, there is often a high level of the hormone DHT, short for dihydrotestosterone, a much more powerful and inflammatory form of testosterone. Prostate enlargement can also be a side effect of drugs used to treat other conditions, such as diuretics, tricyclic antidepressants, opiates, decongestants, and antihistamines. Symptoms improve when treatment shrinks the swelling of the prostate around the urethra.

Prostatitis indicates infection of the prostate, which can include infections by bacteria, yeast, and on rare occasions, viruses. In most cases the infections are short-lived and are resolved by a short course of antibiotics, but some can become chronic or recurring. Unprotected oral sex is a major cause of chronic prostatitis and should be avoided, by both men and women.

Inflammation of the prostate, no matter the cause, can lead to chronic pelvic pain, technically called chronic pelvic pain syndrome. It is often associated with chronic prostatitis and is characterized by pains in the rectum, testicles, penis, low back, and perineum, the area between the rectum and testicles. This pain can vary from day to day and in intensity. Treatment with antibiotics over a long period is often unsuccessful and accompanied by adverse effects.

As men age, inflammation increases throughout their bodies and this contributes to prostate problems. In many cases, chronic or recurring,

---

HOW MANY MEN ARE AFFECTED?

Prostate enlargement becomes more common with age.

- Before age 40: Rare
- After age 60: 60%of men
- After age 80: 80% of men

In more than half of all cases, the degree of enlargement is not severe enough to cause any symptoms.

low-grade infections trigger prostate inflammation, which should resolve once the infection is treated. But sometimes, even after an infection has subsided, the inflammation becomes chronic. It can be turned off with natural substances.

Conventional Treatment

Lifestyle changes can help. These include avoiding caffeine and alcohol, exercising regularly, not drinking fluids before bedtime, and doing Kegel exercises to strengthen the pelvic floor.

Medications for prostate enlargement may include antibiotics to treat an underlying infection, or prostatitis, and these two types of drugs:

Alpha-blockers: While these can reduce symptoms within days or weeks, they do not shrink the prostate or stop its growth. Examples include terazosin (Hytrin), doxazosin (Cardura), and tamsulosin (Flomax). Low blood pressure, dizziness, headache, and a stuffy or runny nose are among the side effects.

5-alpha reductase inhibitors: Also prescribed for hair loss, finasteride (Proscar) and dutasteride (Avodart) shrink the prostate by altering hormone conversion. Side effects include loss of sexual desire and erectile dysfunction.

In extreme cases, the prostate is sometimes removed. Side effects include incontinence and impotence.

My Recommendations

Diet plays a significant role in prostate health. Many foods can worsen inflammation and increase the risk of infections. These include sugar, inflammatory omega-6 oils such as corn, safflower, sunflower, peanut, and soybean oil, used widely in processed and fast foods, and diets high in red meat. Nutrient-dense vegetables, such as broccoli, Brussels sprouts, tomatoes, cauliflower, greens, garlic, onions, cabbage, and kale, reduce inflammation, neutralize free radicals, and lower excessive iron levels, which contribute to problems.

See chapter 3 for how to make a blended drink to easily increase your intake of the most nutritious vegetables. Berries, such as blueberries, blackberries, and raspberries, also reduce prostate inflammation but because of their high sugar content, they should be eaten only in limited amounts. Changing one's diet to an anti-inflammatory one, described in chapter 1, can go a long way in preventing prostate conditions.

🐾 Natural Supplements

▶ Magnesium

Studies have shown that men with prostatitis and prostate cancer have lower prostate tissue magnesium levels than normal. Magnesium is critical for reducing inflammation in tissues and for operation of hundreds of metabolic enzymes. The best way to take magnesium is as magnesium citrate, malate, or as a combination of the two, in a slow-release form.

> ➡ **What to do:** With food, take two caplets daily of Magnesium w/SRT, made by Jigsaw Health. It is a sustained, slow-release magnesium malate which is very well absorbed.

▶ Curcumin and Quercetin

Curcumin and quercetin have very powerful anti-inflammatory properties. In combination, they have been shown to reduce prostate inflammation and inhibit the growth of bacteria within the prostate, which occurs with bacterial prostatitis. For chronic prostate infections, these two supplements work even better when combined with an antibiotic treatment. In one such study, 89 percent of men with chronic bacterial prostatitis treated with antibiotics, curcumin, and quercetin were completely symptom-free after one month, whereas only 27 percent of those treated with antibiotics alone were free of symptoms.

> ➡ **What to do:** For optimum absorption, take 250 mg of each of these, three times daily with meals: a curcumin product called CurcumaSorb, made by Pure Encapsulations, and a

quercetin product called Quercenase, made by Thorne Research. Or, use a powdered form of each and mix with coconut oil or extra virgin olive oil (which can be rather messy).

▶ Prostate Revive

The list of beneficial extracts and nutrients below is quite long. However, they can be found in one prostate formula: Prostate Revive, made by Medix Select. Below I've included approximate dosages and descriptions of key ingredients found in the formula, which is much easier to take than a collection of multiple supplements.

➡ **What to do:** Take one capsule of Prostate Revive, two to three times a day with meals. I would not recommend taking more than three capsules a day. Taking individual supplements below is another option.

▶ Saw Palmetto and Pygeum Extracts

These extracts work by reducing prostate inflammation and by blocking the enzyme that forms the inflammatory form of testosterone, DHT. The blocking of this enzyme, called 5-alpha reductase, is the same action as that of drugs such as Proscar, but the natural products have far fewer side effects and reduce inflammation, which the drugs do not do. Both saw palmetto and pygeum have a long history of effectively reducing inflammatory prostate conditions, and are supported by well-conducted studies that found they are effective over long periods with a very low incidence of side effects. Studies have also found that mixing these two extracts with selenium, lycopene, and stinging nettle extract further enhances their effectiveness.

➡ **What to do:** Take 150 mg of saw palmetto extract and 50 mg of pygeum extract, two to three times daily with meals.

▶ Selenium

The prostate gland concentrates selenium extracted from the blood, indicating its importance in prostate health. Studies have shown that men with prostate enlargement, prostatitis, and prostate cancer have lower prostate selenium levels. Selenium is critical for the proper operation of a vital antioxidant enzyme called glutathione peroxidase.

⮞ **What to do:** Take 100 to 200 mcg a day. Doses higher than 500 mcg a day are associated with damage to the pancreas.

▶ Vitamin D3

Supplementing with vitamin D3 in high doses can improve BPH and reduce the risk of developing the condition. Men destined to have severe prostate enlargement, as well as chronic prostatitis, have a defect in their immune system or are genetically unable to properly utilize vitamin D3. This leads to abnormally low levels of the vitamin, which are associated with inflammation.

⮞ **What to do:** Prostate Revive contains vitamin D3, but I also recommend getting blood levels tested by your doctor and supplementing based on individual needs. The optimum level is between 65 ng/ml and 95 ng/ml. The dose needed depends on the degree of deficiency.

If the level is less than 30 ng/ml, the dose is 10,000 IU of vitamin D3 a day, taken with a meal, for three weeks, and then repeat the blood test. Once blood levels are in the target range, reduce the daily dose to 5,000 IU.

If the blood level is between 35 and 50 ng/ml, I recommend taking 5,000 IU a day for three weeks and then repeating the blood test. If levels are within the optimum range, reduce the dose to 2,000 IU a day. Babies can take 1,000 IU a day and toddlers and small children can take 2,000 IU a day.

▶ Zinc

The prostate gland also has high levels of zinc, which is necessary for proper testosterone function and prostate lubrication of the urethra. Men with BPH have normal to high levels of zinc in their prostate, but those with prostatitis and prostate cancer have very low levels.

➧ **What to do:** Take 10 to 20 mg a day.

▶ <u>**Stinging Nettle Extract**</u>

This extract has powerful anti-inflammatory properties and studies have shown significant benefits in men with prostate conditions, especially BPH and prostatitis.

➧ **What to do:** Take 100 mg, two to three times a day. Higher doses can cause a mucous-like diarrhea.

▶ <u>**Lycopene**</u>

Studies have found that lycopene, which gives tomatoes and watermelons their red pigment, is a powerful anti-inflammatory that is effective in enhancing prostate health.

➧ **What to do:** Take 15 mg a day. Eating tomatoes also helps to protect the prostate.

▶ <u>**Beta-Sitosterol**</u>

A steroid-like compound in plants and saw palmetto, beta-sitosterol has been shown to reduce symptoms of an enlarged prostate, as well as lower cholesterol. Among men taking the supplement, studies have consistently found better urine flow, less residual urine in the bladder after urinating, and fewer trips to the bathroom in the night.

➧ **What to do:** Take 100 mg, twice a day with meals.

Erectile Dysfunction

Most men occasionally experience some difficulty with erections, most often due to stressful situations. In contrast, erectile dysfunction, or "ED," is a persistent problem of not being able to get or maintain an erection. Although it is not a natural or inevitable part of aging, the incidence of ED increases as men get older. It's estimated that between 15 million and 30 million American men suffer from the condition.

Diseases that damage blood vessels restrict blood flow to the penis and, over time, this leads to damage to the mechanism that facilitates an erection. A major cause is atherosclerosis, which is more likely to occur with diabetes. Diabetes can also damage the nerves that enable the penis to function in a normal way. Riding a bicycle with a hard, narrow seat can also cause erectile dysfunction.

RISK FACTORS

These are the most common factors that increase the risk of erectile dysfunction:

- Being over 50 years old
- Cardiovascular disease
- Diabetes
- Elevated blood sugar, or prediabetes
- Excessive drinking
- High blood pressure
- High cholesterol
- Smoking

Studies have shown that 75 percent of men with coronary artery disease, in which plaque blocks blood flow, also have ED. A link between these two conditions may be a deficiency of nitric oxide in the walls of blood vessels, since nitric oxide enables blood vessels to relax, allowing adequate blood flow.

ED is also associated with hypertension, elevated blood fats, obesity, and smoking. Prostate surgery or cancer treatment can damage the nerves in the penis. And sometimes, ED is a side effect of blood pressure-lowering drugs, pain medications, antidepressants, or antihistamines.

☙ Conventional Treatment

Treating any underlying conditions, especially if the right lifestyle changes are made, can help to prevent or reverse ED. Otherwise, ED drugs are a common treatment, including sildenafil citrate (Viagra), vardenafil HCl (Levitra), and tadalafil (Cialis). Side effects can include headaches, muscle aches, a stuffy nose, and flushing, and the drugs may have serious complications such as increased risk for heart attack and vision loss.

A vacuum pump is an alternative to drugs. By creating a vacuum around erectile tissue, it triggers an erection. In extreme cases, penile implants can be done, but these are rare.

👍 My Recommendations

As with most medical conditions, a healthy diet, exercise, avoiding excessive or chronic stress, and getting restful sleep all play a role in preventing ED. The problem is more likely to occur with a diet that accelerates atherosclerosis: one that is high in sugar, especially high fructose corn syrup; rich in inflammatory omega-6 fats, such as corn, safflower, sunflower, peanut, and soybean oils widely used in processed foods; deficient in healthy omega-3 fats found in fish, nuts, and seeds; and low in vegetables. Chapter 1 lays out an anti-inflammatory way of eating that solves these problems.

Exposure to pesticides, herbicides, and fungicides increases levels of estrogen and lowers levels of testosterone and this, too, can interfere with the ability to attain an erection. Eating organic foods and avoiding toxic grooming products can decrease exposure to testosterone-disrupting toxins.

🐇 Natural Supplements
▶ Carnitine

Studies have found that carnitine, a nutrient found chiefly in red meat, can improve erectile function, sometimes even better than testosterone treatment. In supplements, it comes in different forms—L-carnitine, acetyl-L-carnitine, and propionyl-L-carnitine—and all are effective. In one study, a combination of acetyl-L-carnitine, propionyl-L-carnitine, and Viagra worked better than the drug alone. Most studies have used two grams daily of carnitine, in divided doses.

➡ **What to do:** Take two capsules, 500 mg each, two to three times daily, 30 minutes before meals.

▶ Niacin

A study of 160 men with ED and atherosclerosis found that niacin supplements significantly improved erectile function, with best results seen in those with severe or moderate ED. The main side effects of niacin are itching and stomach upset, and sustained-release forms are associated with a high risk of liver damage.

➡ **What to do:** I do not strongly favor niacin for ED but if you want to try it, take 500 mg at bedtime and see how you tolerate it, and slowly build up to 1,000 to 1,500 mg daily over a two-week period.

▶ Panax Ginseng

Online, some people call red or Korean ginseng "herbal Viagra." Studies have found that taking 900 to 1,000 mg, three times a day with meals, improved erectile function, but in most cases, the improvement was not dramatic. This particular species of ginseng appears to enhance blood flow to the penis, by increasing nitric oxide in penile blood vessels, and to increase penile rigidity and function. It does not increase testosterone levels. Panax ginseng can cause nervousness and insomnia, especially if taken in the evening. In general, it improves stamina and memory and elevates one's mood.

➡ **What to do:** Take 900 to 1,000 mg, three times daily with meals.

▶ DHEA

Short for dehydroepiandrosterone, DHEA is a natural compound used by our bodies to make testosterone and estrogen. ED is much more common in men with low DHEA levels, which can be measured with a blood test. Most studies show only moderate effects on ED.

➡ **What to do:** Take 50 mg a day, with or without food.

▶ Zinc

Zinc is an essential mineral used by the body to produce testosterone. It is estimated that 45 percent of males over age 60 are deficient in zinc, which is found mainly in meats, fish, and nuts. It's a good idea to get a zinc RBC (red blood cell) test from your doctor.

> ➡ **What to do:** After age 60, take 15 to 30 mg a day, depending on the level of your deficiency. Zinc Picolinate, made by Thorne Research, is a good product.

▶ L-Arginine and Pycnogenol

L-arginine is a naturally occurring amino acid, and Pycnogenol (pronounced "pick-gnaw-ju-nol") is a special extract from French maritime pine bark. Both increase production of nitric oxide, thereby improving blood flow to the penis, but each works differently. Together, they work more efficiently than either alone. In studies of men with ED, the combination enabled erections in 80 percent of men after two months, and in 92.5 percent after three months.

> ➡ **What to do:** Take 1,000 mg of L-arginine and 100 mg of Pycnogenol, three times daily.

▶ Vitamin D3

In addition to being a nutrient, vitamin D3 is also a hormone and it increases testosterone levels. Low vitamin D levels are typical among men suffering from ED.

> ➡ **What to do:** Before taking vitamin D3 as a supplement, blood vitamin D3 levels should be tested. This is a common test. The optimum level is between 65 ng/ml and 95 ng/ml. The dose depends on the degree of deficiency.
>
> If the level is less than 30 ng/ml, the dose is 10,000 IU of vitamin D3 a day, taken with a meal, for three weeks, and then repeat the blood test. Once blood levels are in the target range, reduce the daily dose to 5,000 IU.

If the blood level is between 35 and 50 ng/ml, I recommend taking 5,000 IU a day for three weeks and then repeating the blood test. If levels are within the optimum range, reduce the dose to 2,000 IU a day.

▶ Other Beneficial Extracts

Some studies have found that regular use of other herbal extracts, for anywhere from weeks to months, can also improve ED. These include 120 mg of ginkgo biloba, twice daily; 20 mg of vinpocetine, once or twice daily; and 1.5 to 3 grams daily of maca. Combinations of these can work better than one extract alone, and they are sometimes found in supplement formulas designed for men.

▶ Hyperbaric Oxygen Therapy (HBOT)

In certain cases of erectile dysfunction, the penile nerves are damaged. In such instances, there is some evidence that HBOT can improve the condition, as it can help to restore nerve function.

CHAPTER 7

Women's Health

» Menopausal Symptoms
» Menstrual Difficulties
» Sexual Difficulties
» Urinary Tract Infections
» Varicose Veins

Menopausal Symptoms

Technically, menopause means that a woman has not had a menstrual period for at least 12 months. However, the term is generally used to describe a duration of several years when hormone levels are gradually changing and, in some women, produce uncomfortable symptoms, such as hot flashes, mood swings, sleep disturbances, and pain during intercourse.

Medically, this stage is more accurately called "perimenopause." The prefix "peri" means "around," meaning the time around menopause in this case. Symptoms can occur in any order. For example, a woman may easily get tired or feel depressed for months or even years before hot flashes appear.

⚕ Conventional Treatment

Hormone replacement therapy, or HRT, was popular until a large clinical trial found that it increased risk for stroke and heart disease. Since then, these findings have been disputed, but the treatment remains controversial. Other studies have found that the most commonly prescribed, artificial form of estrogen also increases risks for breast and ovarian cancers. As an alternative to HRT, conventional doctors often prescribe antidepressants, which do not address hormonal fluctuations, have side effects, and pose many other risks.

👍 My Recommendations

Hormone therapy can be safe and effective but the conventional approach is incorrect and dangerous. There are three forms of estrogen in the body: estradiol, estrone, and estriol. Estradiol is the most powerful and, in excess, can trigger inflammation, yet the most common HRT prescription is Premarin, an artificial form of inflammatory estradiol.

Estrone and estriol are much weaker forms of estrogen and reduce breast cancer risk, instead of increasing it. Physicians trained in natural hormone replacement usually use estriol. In addition, they run tests to determine individual needs for estrogen and other hormones to maintain a healthy balance.

> **MENOPAUSE FACTS**
>
> - The average age of menopause is 51.
> - Most often, it occurs between the ages of 45 and 55, but can occur earlier or later.
> - Women who undergo a hysterectomy may experience more severe menopausal symptoms after the surgery, even if they are much younger.

For any woman experiencing uncomfortable symptoms, I recommend working with a physician who is well-versed in nutrition and natural hormone therapy, and getting a comprehensive panel of hormone tests, which includes measuring all three forms of estrogen. Then, a natural hormone prescription can be customized.

Not all women need any type of hormone replacement. Eating plenty of vegetables, especially cruciferous ones, reduces inflammation that has been found to be responsible for a number of menopause symptoms, such as hot flashes, mood swings, depression, anxiety, and sleep disturbances. And, vegetables contain nutrients with weak and beneficial estrogenic effects.

Although soy is a source of plant estrogen, I do not recommend soy products, especially soymilk, as these typically also contain substances that are toxic to the brain, such as glutamate (see chapter 2), aluminum, and fluoride. Soy also elevates an enzyme called aromatase, which increases breast cancer growth.

Pesticides and herbicides, which disrupt hormones, should be avoided by eating organic foods. And, steer clear of pro-inflammatory omega-6 fats, such as corn, safflower, sunflower, peanut, and soybean oils in processed foods. Instead, choose fish, extra virgin olive oil, and coconut oil, which are all good sources of anti-inflammatory, healthy fats. Chapter 1 describes my recommended diet.

Natural Supplements

▶ Quercetin

A nutrient found in plants, quercetin has weak estrogenic effects and can assist in reducing menopausal symptoms. It is also a powerful inhibitor of breast cancer. I recommend Quercenase, made by Thorne Research.

> ➡ **What to do:** Take one 250 mg capsule, two to three times a day with meals.

▶ Curcumin

This extract of the curry spice turmeric has been shown to protect against harmful estrogenic effects of pesticides and herbicides and is anti-inflammatory. In addition, it has powerful antioxidant, antibacterial, antiviral, and cancer-inhibiting effects. Curcumin is not well absorbed, unless it is mixed with oils or in a supplement that is specially designed to be easily broken down, such as CurcumaSorb, made by Pure Encapsulations.

➡ **What to do:** Take 250 mg, three times a day with meals.

▶ **Black Cohosh**

Studies suggest that in a significant number of women, a black cohosh extract can relieve the symptoms of menopause, especially flushing and hot flashes, and helps prevent osteoporosis. There have been rare cases of liver injury associated with its use. It comes in tablets, capsules, and as a tincture.

➡ **What to do:** Take 540 mg a day with food.

▶ **Green and White Teas**

Green and white tea can reduce some of the symptoms of menopause and can help strengthen bones. White tea can be had three times a day, or take a concentrated green tea supplement, such as Teavigo, a standardized extract that is an ingredient in many supplement brands.

➡ **What to do:** Take 100 mg of Teavigo, once a day with food.

▶ **DHA**

This is one of the chief omega-3 oils in fish. Because many of the symptoms of menopause are inflammatory in nature, DHA can reduce inflammation and symptoms. Flaxseed oil is another source of omega-3 fats but it is not the same form as the DHA in fish oil and does not produce identical benefits. If you prefer a vegan source, DHA from algae is available in supplements.

➡ **What to do:** Take at least 1,000 mg a day of DHA, from fish oil or algae.

Menstrual Difficulties

Menstrual cycles vary in length, frequency, and intensity. The average length between periods is 28 days and the average length of a period is three to five days, but these can differ substantially from one woman to another. Tracking when periods occur, how long they last, and any notable symptoms is helpful for detecting changes, because it is the changes in an individual's pattern that may indicate a problem.

The degree and type of discomfort also varies for each individual. Severe symptoms can be a sign of an underlying condition, such as uterine fibroids or endometriosis—growth of uterine tissue outside the uterus. Often, these don't pose a health threat but the symptoms can be debilitating.

Conventional Treatment

Lifestyle changes, including regular exercise, a nutritious diet, and adequate sleep, can all help to make a woman's monthly cycle less eventful. Since menstrual periods are a natural part of life, rather than a disease, there is no specific drug to treat symptoms. However, doctors sometimes prescribe birth control pills to regulate periods or antidepressants to dull the effects of symptoms, despite their risks and side effects. When severe discomfort or pain stems from uterine fibroids or endometriosis, surgery is often an option.

A cessation of periods, or amenorrhea, can be the result of extreme exercise and/or extreme dieting, or it can indicate the beginnings of anorexia nervosa. And, various monthly discomforts can result from or be intensified by a poor diet that disrupts normal hormonal function.

My Recommendations

A healthy diet consists of 5 to 10 servings of mostly vegetables and some fruits, moderate meat intake of 4 to 6 ounces a day, carbohydrates that are not sugary or starchy, beverages without fluoride, and wholesome, fresh foods rather than those that are processed or high in sugar. Fats should be healthy, anti-inflammatory omega-3 oils from fish, coconut oil, and extra virgin olive oil, instead of pro-inflammatory ones, such as corn, safflower, sunflower, peanut, soybean, and canola oils in processed foods.

Fluoride can trigger menstrual symptoms and impairs reproductive health. Fluoride sources include fluoridated drinking water, black tea, fluoridated mouthwash and toothpaste, and fluoride treatments at the dentist.

UNCOMFORTABLE MENSTRUAL SYMPTOMS	
• Bloating	• Mood swings
• Breast tenderness	• No periods
• Cramps	• Pain
• Headaches	• Spotting
• Heavy periods	• Water retention
• Insomnia	• Weight gain
• Irregular periods	

Obesity doubles the chances of menstrual problems, most likely because of increased inflammation and insulin resistance, a condition in which sugars and starches can no longer be metabolized normally, leading to elevated levels of glucose in the blood. A healthy diet can normalize weight as well as support healthy hormonal balance.

Natural Supplements
▶ Chaste Berry Extract

Studies show that chaste berry, also called vitex (short for the herb's Latin name, *Vitex agnus-castus*), is highly effective in preventing and treating menstrual irregularities, cramps, breast tenderness and pain, and anxiety and depression associated with PMS. Equally important, it has a high degree of safety.

> ➡ **What to do:** Take 400 mg, two to three times a day, with or without food. The herb's effectiveness increases over time and it may take four to six weeks to achieve optimum relief.

▶ Korean Red Ginseng

Several studies have shown that it can significantly reduce menstrual irregularities, cramping, pain, and other symptoms. In addition, this extract has another very important benefit: it blocks the damaging effect of bisphenol A (BPA), a hormone-disrupting toxin in plastics and linings of cans. A good brand is Imperial Elixir Korean Red Ginseng, made by Ginco International.

> ➠ **What to do:** Take 600 mg, twice a day with meals. For more severe problems, take the same dose three times a day.

▶ Magnesium Malate

Magnesium relieves uterine cramping, reduces inflammation, calms the nervous system, and relieves anxiety and depression. Take a slow-release form of magnesium malate. I recommend Magnesium w/SRT, made by Jigsaw Health.

> ➠ **What to do:** Take two caplets, twice a day with meals.

▶ Ginger and Zinc Picolinate

Studies have found that a combination of ginger and zinc significantly reduces uterine cramping, and ginger reduces heavy menstrual bleeding. Ginger can also lower blood sugar, which may be a benefit for some people but can be a problem for those with hypoglycemia.

> ➠ **What to do:** Take 1,100 mg of ginger, three times a day with meals, and 30 mg of zinc daily, with or without a meal. For zinc, I recommend Zing Picolinate, made by Thorne Research.

▶ Omega-3 Oils

Omega-3 oils are beneficial because they are very anti-inflammatory. I recommend Carlson's lemon- or orange-flavored liquid fish oil with EPA and DHA.

> ➠ **What to do:** Take two teaspoons of the oil, two to three times a day with a meal.

Urinary Tract Infections

Second only to colds and flu as a reason for seeing a doctor, urinary tract infections are much more common among women than men, and they are somewhat misunderstood. Many consider that the urinary tract consists only of the tube through which urine is excreted, but it also includes the bladder and kidneys. If an infection spreads to the kidneys, it can pose serious risk, especially for an older person who is less resistant to infection. Low-grade, smoldering infections, and recurrent infections pose the greatest danger, and can result in kidney failure.

Conventional Treatment

Because urinary tract infections are usually bacterial, they can respond to antibiotics. However, repeated use of antibiotics or not completing a course of antibiotics can lead to antibiotic resistance, making some no longer effective. Consequently, alternative antibiotics may need to be prescribed.

Newer studies show that bacteria can hide by sealing off in an impenetrable biofilm and sticking to the lining of the bladder, kidneys, or urethra, becoming inaccessible to antibiotics. Infections may continue or recur.

Whenever possible, prevention is the best strategy. These habits can help:

- Going to the bathroom more often, and always after sex
- Drinking unsweetened cranberry juice every day
- Drinking more water to help eliminate bacteria
- Not using internal feminine hygiene products
- Not using spermicides with diaphragms

👍 My Recommendations

Some of the compounds in white and green tea, and in many vegetables, such as broccoli, Brussels sprouts, kale, and garlic, can prevent and suppress bacterial growth. In contrast, high-sugar diets promote urinary tract and yeast infections. All sugars do this, including cane sugar, sucrose, dextrose, glucose, fructose, and honey. Inflammatory omega-6 oils, such as corn, safflower, sunflower, peanut, soybean, and canola oils can worsen urinary tract infections. And fluoride should be avoided, because it can interfere with natural immunity and promotes inflammation.

> **SYMPTOMS OF A URINARY TRACT INFECTION**
>
> If a urinary tract infection spreads to the kidneys, it can cause fever or chills. More common symptoms include:
> - A burning feeling when urinating
> - Dark, cloudy, and/or strong-smelling urine
> - Feeling the urge to urinate often, but little comes out
> - Pressure or pain in the lower back or abdomen
> - Feeling tired

While it is best to avoid antibiotics as a first treatment choice, studies have shown that combining natural supplements with antibiotics makes them much more successful in eliminating the infection. If antibiotics are taken, probiotics should be taken with the medication and for at least two weeks afterwards, to replenish beneficial bacteria. This will reduce antibiotic side effects and help prevent future infections. For details on using probiotics, see the "Digestion" section on "Diarrhea."

🫒 Natural Supplements

▶ Cranberry Juice or Extract

A number of studies show that compounds found in cranberries significantly prevent and suppress the growth of bacteria in the urinary tract. Cranberry extracts are a good choice because they don't contain the sugar usually found in cranberry juices. If you prefer drinking cranberry, I recommend a product called FruitFast Cranberry Juice Concentrate, made by Brownwood Acres, which contains the beneficial compounds with reduced sugar. A good extract is Standardized Cranberry, made by NOW Foods, which also contains uva ursi, which kills yeast and dissolves biofilm that seals in bacteria, and grape seed extract.

➡ **What to do:** Take 1 tablespoon of FruitFast Cranberry Juice Concentrate, two to three times a day, or 1 capsule of NOW Foods Standardized Cranberry, three times a day with meals.

▶ Luteolin

It has been shown to reduce the adherence of bacteria to kidney and bladder cells and inhibit biofilm formation around bacteria, which all help to clear bacteria from the urinary tract.

➡ **What to do:** Take 100 to 200 mg, three times a day with meals.

▶ Quercetin

Studies show that this plant nutrient can powerfully inhibit biofilm formation by one or more types of bacteria that can infect the urinary tract, thereby making them easier to eliminate. I recommend Quercenase, a well-absorbed form made by Thorne Research.

➡ **What to do:** Take one to two capsules, three times a day with meals.

▶ Curcumin

Studies have shown that curcumin, an extract from the curry spice turmeric, is another powerful inhibitor of biofilm formation. It also inhibits the motility of bacteria, meaning it impairs their ability to swim. And, it reduces inflammation in infected tissues. I recommend an absorbable form, CurcumaSorb, made by Pure Encapsulations.

➡ **What to do:** Take one to two capsules, three times a day with meals.

▶ D-Mannose

This is a special type of sugar molecule that fights infections in a different way. After you take D-mannose, the kidneys secrete it in high concentrations into the bladder. Bacteria cling to the D-mannose and get washed out. It is particularly effective at getting rid of E. coli, the most common infecting organism in urinary tract infections. D-mannose is best used at the first sign of an infection.

➡ **What to do:** Take 500 mg of D-mannose powder mixed with 6 ounces of water, every two hours for five days. This frequent dosing maintains high levels of D-mannose in the urine and flushes out bacteria.

▶ Hyperbaric Oxygen Therapy (HBOT)

There is good evidence that HBOT can aid in the clearance of bacterial infections of the bladder, especially in cases of resistant and recurrent infections. The best results are seen when antibiotics are combined with HBOT.

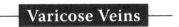

Varicose Veins

More common among women than men, varicose veins are swollen, twisted veins that are often visible just under the skin in the legs, but they can also occur in other parts of the body—as hemorrhoids, for example. Hemorrhoids can rupture, causing rectal bleeding or blood-streaked bowel movements. So-called spider veins are usually an early sign of further, more serious, problems in the future.

To keep blood flowing toward the heart, veins naturally have valves to control the flow. When the valves become weak, blood flow slows down and can pool, leading to swollen veins.

The walls of the veins also become leaky, allowing serum from the blood to seep into the tissues, resulting in swelling called edema. Pushing on the swollen tissue can leave it indented for several seconds, called pitting edema. More severe cases can include skin discoloration and ulceration, and is accompanied by chronic inflammation within the veins.

Conventional Treatment

Varicose veins that develop during pregnancy sometimes resolve on their own, but in other situations, they persist and may or may not require treatment. Sometimes, they cause pain or throbbing, or may lead to sores developing in the area, because of restricted blood flow. But often, they are only a cosmetic problem. Straining during bowel movements is a common cause of hemorrhoids.

Avoiding standing for long periods, elevating legs when sitting or sleeping, and wearing compression stockings are all helpful strategies to prevent or contain the condition. Treatments to eliminate varicose veins include destruction of the veins with injected medications, lasers, radio frequency, or surgery.

RISK FACTORS FOR VARICOSE VEINS
Varicose veins are more likely to affect:
• Women
• Older people
• Those who do not exercise regularly
• Anyone who is obese
• Women who are pregnant
• Those with a family history of the condition

Weakness of the valves in deep veins can lead to a clotting of the veins, technically called thrombosis. This can be quite dangerous if clots break loose and lodge in deep veins that lead to the lungs, as in the case of a pulmonary embolism. However, this is not a danger with the more superficial veins.

My Recommendations

Heredity sometimes plays a role but other factors are always present and can be controlled. Recent studies indicate that low-grade inflammation and free radicals, which cause internal damage much like rusting, are also involved. The supplements below and nutrients found in a multivitamin and mineral supplement, such as Extend Core, made by Vitamin Research Products, play an important part in protecting one from weakened veins.

An anti-inflammatory diet, described in chapter 1, helps to strengthen walls of blood vessels and reduce the risk of varicose veins and blood clots. It includes fruits, vegetables, a moderate amount of protein, healthy fats, and purified water.

Natural Supplements

▶ Hesperidin and Diosmin

The combination of these two extracts has been extensively tested and shown to significantly improve varicose veins and prevent their progression. I recommend a product called DiosVein, made by Swanson Health Products, which contains 500 mg of diosmin and 100 mg of hesperidin per capsule.

> ➡ **What to do:** Take two capsules, three times a day, with or without meals.

▶ Vitamin C

Vitamin C plays an essential role in strengthening veins, and decreases inflammation and free radical damage, which is much like internal rusting. This reduces swelling and leakiness of the veins. The most potent product is Lypo-Spheric Vitamin C, made by LivOn Labs, which comes in a gel form in 1,000-mg packets. Buffered vitamin C is also a good form.

> ➡ **What to do:** Take 1,000 mg of Lypo-Spheric Vitamin C, twice a day, or 250 mg of buffered vitamin C, three times a day.

▶ Curcumin

An extract from the curry spice turmeric, curcumin has been shown to strengthen blood vessels, reduce vein leakiness, neutralize free radicals, and promote healing. CurcumaSorb, made by Pure Encapsulations, is a well-absorbed form.

➡ **What to do:** Take 250 mg, three times a day with meals.

▶ **Lysine**

An amino acid, lysine plays a major role in reinforcing connective tissue that makes veins strong.

➡ **What to do:** Take 500 mg, three times a day, 30 minutes before meals.

▶ **Magnesium**

Magnesium is important for maintaining blood flow inside blood vessels, substantially reducing risk of harmful clots, reducing inflammation, and neutralizing free radicals that cause internal rusting. A slow-release magnesium malate is best, found in Magnesium s/SRT, made by Jigsaw Health.

➡ **What to do:** Take two caplets, twice a day, at breakfast and dinner.

The Importance of Good Nutrition

A number of the health problems women face are associated with an improper diet and the use of certain processed foods and drinks. It must be appreciated that certain conditions, such as menopause, are natural phenomena associated with an ending of the period of fertility. These natural states can become pathological when life-disturbing symptoms become dominant. The same is true during the period of fertility for the younger woman. Diet can play a vital role in reproductive health.

Likewise, many other conditions, such as infections, can also be altered by diet. A poor diet, filled with omega-6 oils, sugar, artificial sweeteners, grains, soy foods, and red meats can increase one's risk, while a healthy diet can protect against many of these problems.

The foundation of good health is based on the knowledge that our bodies are always changing—cells are reproducing, replacing dying cells; tissues are being altered to accommodate environmental changes; and organs require a constant supply of specialized nutrients for their function and protection. We often think of our bodies as unchanging and this causes us to ignore the importance of a constant supply of essential nutrients.

CHAPTER 8

Pain

Back Pain and Sciatica

Pain in the back, especially the lower back, affects nearly everyone at some time. In most cases, it goes away without treatment in a few days or weeks. Most often, it stems from an injury, which can include doing extra work in the garden, cleaning out an attic or garage, playing sports on the weekend, or receiving a sudden jolt, such as in a car accident or fall. Symptoms can range from sore muscles to shooting pains, and from difficulty moving to being unable to stand straight. Back pain that lasts more than two weeks is classified as chronic back pain and can persist for years. In most cases, the pain varies in intensity—with good days and bad days.

The spine is a column of bones and intervening joints, with more than 30 bones held in place by tendons and ligaments, separated by discs that act as cushions. Muscles of the back attach to the spine bones, enabling movement of the body. The spinal cord, which contains more than 30 pairs of nerves, is housed in an open channel within the upper spine down to the upper lumbar spine. When the structure is overstressed or injured, a disc may become compressed, bulge, or rupture, putting pressure on a nerve and causing extreme pain.

BACK PAIN FACTS

According to the National Institute of Arthritis and Musculoskeletal and Skin Diseases, back pain is more common among people who:

- Are physically unfit
- Are overweight
- Are older
- Lift heavy objects at work
- Repetitively perform twisting, pulling, or pushing movements at work
- Sit all day and have poor posture

Sciatica is a different pattern of pain. The largest and longest nerve in the body, the sciatic nerve runs from the lower spine, down the back of the thigh, behind the knee, and down the back of the calf, all the way through the sole of the foot to the toes. At the spinal end, it is actually a combination of five nerves which become one, and at the largest point, it is about as wide as a man's thumb. As the nerve travels down the back of the leg, it splits into several nerves that provide sensation and signals that enable the muscles to work.

When irritated, the sciatic nerve can cause shooting or burning, sharp pain, which usually feels better while walking or lying down, and worse when standing or sitting. In many cases, the pain begins as a deep aching in the buttocks region and can extend only a short distance, or down the entire course of the nerve. Tingling, numbness, or a feeling of pressure may also occur. Symptoms usually appear on only one side of the body. Most cases are caused by compression of a nerve at the spinal end of the sciatic nerve.

Both back pain and sciatica share underlying mechanisms that cause the sensation of pain: inflammation and excitotoxicity (see chapter 2) at the site of the compressed nerve. Reducing these helps to relieve pain.

👌 Conventional Treatment for Back Pain

Over-the-counter pain relievers are the most common remedy, but can lead to dependence and stomach bleeding. These and prescription pain relievers generally aim to reduce inflammation, which allows the body to heal itself.

A combination of cold compresses or ice for a few days, followed by heat compresses or a heating pad, are common remedies, although they don't always eliminate pain. Chiropractic spine manipulation and

> **DANGEROUS SCIATICA SYMPTOMS**
>
> Immediate medical attention is required if any of these symptoms appear:
> - Numbness in one or both legs or feet
> - Weakness in the legs or feet
> - Loss of sensation in one or both legs
> - Loss of control of the bowel or bladder

prescribed exercises are also used. However, staying in bed, while it might be tempting, can make the pain worse.

In severe situations of chronic back pain, surgery to relieve pressure on nerves, or to sever nerve fibers to prevent transmission of pain, are treatments of last resort. There is no guarantee of success.

👌 Conventional Treatment for Sciatica

Sometimes, sciatica goes away without any treatment and in many cases there is no known cause. However, sciatica can also be a sign of a ruptured disc or other injury, such as a fractured pelvis, or a narrowing of the spinal canal, which then exerts pressure on the nerve. Treatment, which may include exercise, medications, and/or surgery, depends upon the diagnosis.

👍 My Recommendations

Newer studies show that inflammation and excitotoxicity play major roles in acute and chronic spinal pain. Excitotoxicity means levels of a neurotransmitter, called glutamate, are excessively high and are causing damage, including pain.

Glutamate can come from two sources: the body makes it, in excess at the site of pain, and it is also a food additive, for example, in MSG (monosodium glutamate). When there is excess glutamate from diet, on top of excess glutamate generated by the body, it magnifies the problem and the pain. When combined with inflammation, it's much like pouring multiple fuels onto a burning fire, making it rage all the more.

The right diet can calm the inferno in two ways: by reducing internal inflammation and excitotoxicity, and by reducing excess body fat where necessary. For anyone who is overweight, reducing weight reduces stress on all joints, including the spine. While this may seem obvious, it's often overlooked. In addition, belly fat generates inflammation, which subsides when belly fat is lost. Chapter 1 outlines an anti-inflammatory diet. Chapter 2 explains excitotoxins and how to avoid them, especially by not eating food additives with glutamate. And chapter 3 makes it easy to develop a vital habit: eating significantly more nutritious vegetables every day, by making a vegetable drink. Vegetables are vital to calm inflammation and excitotoxicity.

Fluoride is another cause of chronic back pain. Over many years, it can accumulate in bones, causing spinal bones to overgrow, narrowing the channel that houses the spinal cord and nerves. Fluoride accumulation can also contribute to bone spurs that can impinge on spinal nerves and cause pain. It is important to avoid all sources of fluoride, such as fluoridated drinking water, fluoridated toothpaste and mouthwash, foods and drinks that contain fluoride, and fluoride dental treatments.

Exercise is Vital

In addition to the right diet, exercise is vital to strengthen the muscles that support the spine, which weaken with a sedentary lifestyle and predispose one to injury from minor stress on the back during everyday activities. Improper lifting is also a common cause of back pain and sciatica.

Studies of large numbers of people with chronic back pain, using MRI scans, found that those with the most pain had the smallest muscles supporting the spine; those muscles were atrophied from lack of use. Building up these muscles with exercises dramatically reduced the pain and, in many cases, cured it.

Both back muscles and abdominal muscles need to be strong to support the spine and protect it from injury during relatively minor exertion. There are many exercises to build up these muscles but these are two simple ones I recommend for back pain:

LEG LIFTS

Lie on the floor with knees bent at a 90-degree angle, hands by your sides. Slowly lift your legs, keeping the knees bent, as high as you can without straining or using your arms, and then slowly lower to the starting position. The movement should be controlled, without using your arms or momentum, and you should feel abdominal muscles working. Repeat 10 to 12 times, or as many as you can. If you're able to, rest and do one or two more sets of 10 to 12 repetitions. If this is painful, don't do it. Go to http://homegym-exercises.com/bent_knee_leg_raise_lying.html to view a video example.

BACK EXTENSION

This can be done at home using an exercise ball, an inexpensive item that is available wherever fitness gadgets are sold. To start, lie on the ball, face down, so that your hips are on top of the ball and your upper body is draped over it. With your elbows bent and one hand on top of the other in front of your chest, push your hips into the ball and extend your upper body upward, slowly, and return to the starting position. Repeat 10 to 12 times, or as many as you can. If you're able to, rest and do one or two more sets of 10 to 12 repetitions. If this is painful, don't do it. Go to www.exrx.net/ WeightExercises/ErectorSpinae/BWHyperextensionBallArms Crossed.html to view a video example.

✒️ Natural Supplements for Back Pain

While supplements are not generally needed for controlling most back pain, in many cases they are helpful by reducing inflammation and excitotoxicity. Here are the ones I would most recommend.

▶ DHA from Fish Oil

Increasing your omega-3 oil intake reduces inflammation everywhere in your body and can significantly reduce all forms of pain. Fish oil contains two key components, EPA and DHA. The DHA component has been shown to reduce inflammation and excitotoxicity, the best of all worlds. DHA is available as a separate supplement. As another option, DHA is available in a brain health formula with other ingredients that reduce excitotoxicity, called Keralex, made by Medix Select.

➡ **What to do:** Take 500 to 1,000 mg of DHA, twice a day. Or, take two capsules of Keralex, three to four times a day.

▶ Curcumin and Quercetin

Both curcumin and quercetin reduce inflammation in different ways that are complementary, so they work well together. With both, it's important to take products that are formulated to be well absorbed, such as CurcumaSorb, made by Pure Encapsulations, and Quercenase, made by Thorne Research. Both contain 250 mg per capsule.

➡ **What to do:** Take two capsules of CurcumaSorb and one to two capsules of Quercenase, three times a day with meals.

▶ Chondroitin Sulfate

This is a naturally occurring compound that is essential for the maintenance of cartilage in joints. A number of studies have shown that it can improve inflammatory conditions that damage cartilage, such as a lumbar disc. Relief usually begins within a few weeks and continued use may prevent a relapse of disc degeneration. Chondroitin sulfate does not interfere with medications.

➡ **What to do:** Take 600 mg, three times a day with meals.

▶ Buffered Vitamin C

An interesting study, reported in the *Journal of Neurosurgery*, demonstrated a complete reversal of a ruptured lumbar disc in a patient taking high doses of vitamin C. The vitamin is essential for maintenance of disc cartilage, strengthens lumbar tendons and ligaments, and reduces inflammation. Smoking, a habit that is associated with a high incidence of ruptured lumbar disc and low back pain, causes a severe loss of vitamin C.

➡ **What to do:** Take a buffered form of vitamin C (described as such on labels), 500 to 1,000 mg, three times a day between meals. Never take high doses of vitamin C with food because it dramatically increases iron absorption, potentially to excessive levels.

Natural Supplements for Sciatica

Take curcumin and quercetin, as for back pain above. DHA from fish oil may also help, as it reduces inflammation. These are other supplements, which work together in a complementary way and can help reduce inflammation, excitotoxicity, and pain of sciatica.

▶ Hesperidin

Hesperidin is a flavonoid, a therapeutic plant compound, found in higher concentrations in oranges. A number of studies have shown that hesperidin reduces inflammation, inhibits excitotoxicity, and reduces depression, a major contributor to chronic pain.

➡ **What to do:** Take one to two 500 mg capsules, three times a day with meals.

▶ Apigenin

Several studies have shown that apigenin, a flavonoid found in high concentrations in celery, parsley, apples, and chamomile, can reduce pain. Aside from taking it as a supplement, you can ingest apigenin by drinking chamomile tea. A good concentrated extract is Apigenin, made by Swanson Health Products, which contains 50 mg per capsule.

➡ **What to do:** Take two capsules (100 mg), three times a day with meals.

▶ Luteolin
Also a plant flavonoid, luteolin has also been shown to calm specific inflammation-generating mechanisms and reduce pain levels.

➡ **What to do:** Take 100 mg, three times a day.

▶ R-lipoic acid
This is a strong antioxidant and anti-inflammatory that is very effective for diabetic nerve pain and may help relieve sciatica.

➡ **What to do:** Take 100 to 200 mg with each meal.

▶ Acetyl-L Carnitine with Vinpocetine
Both of these natural substances help repair nerves, improve their function, and significantly reduce nerve pain. Vinpocetine also improves blood flow to damaged nerves, which promotes healing. A product called Cresceo-ALC, made by Medix Select, contains this combination with 750 mg of acetyl-L-carnitine and 15 mg of vinpocetine in each capsule.

➡ **What to do:** Take one capsule, two to three times a day, 30 minutes before meals.

▶ Hyperbaric Oxygen Therapy (HBOT)
Several studies have shown that HBOT treatments can stimulate healing of damaged nerves. Therefore, it may help with sciatica. Given the time and expense involved in obtaining HBOT, other treatments should be tried first.

Carpal Tunnel Syndrome

A condition that develops from overuse of the wrist, carpal tunnel syndrome manifests as pain, numbness, and weakness in the hand and wrist which radiates up the arm. The carpal tunnel is at the base of the hand and houses tendons and a major nerve, the median nerve, which transmits signals that enable the hand, thumb, and most of the fingers (all but the little and ring fingers) to feel and move.

In this condition, the tunnel narrows, putting pressure on the median nerve. And that pressure causes the symptoms, which can be debilitating. On occasion, the radiating pain up the arm can resemble that of an impending heart attack. Carpal tunnel numbness frequently occurs during sleep because of the position of the hands. Holding the hands in a flexed position can precipitate the pain and numbness. Repetitive use of computers and tools that vibrate, such as weed-eaters, jack-hammers, and leaf blowers can cause carpal tunnel syndrome and precipitate an attack.

Conventional Treatment

Resting the wrist for at least two weeks, immobilizing it in a splint, and avoiding activity that can aggravate the condition are first lines of treatment. Other medical conditions, such as arthritis, hypothyroidism, or diabetes, may underlie carpal tunnel syndrome, and where these exist, they should be diagnosed and treated.

Over-the-counter pain relievers are sometimes taken but have risks for longer-term use. Where the condition is not chronic, diuretics (water pills) or corticosteroids may be used to help to reduce swelling. Or, steroids mixed with lidocaine, a local anesthetic, may be injected into the wrist to reduce pressure on the nerve. Exercise can also help.

Where carpal tunnel syndrome lasts for more than six months, surgery may be done to cut the carpal ligament. If done correctly, it has a high degree of success and most patients have complete or near-complete recovery. Recurrence after surgery is unusual.

👍 My Recommendations

In many cases, the problem can be reversed simply by changing a few work habits or by avoiding vibrating work tools. People doing a lot of computer work often suffer from this malady either from their hand position or from resting their wrist on a hard surface or edge. Padding these surfaces can help a lot. In early cases of carpal tunnel, I have found that stretching the area of the wrist and kneading the skin over the carpal tunnel can occasionally cure the problem. Also, running cold water or applying a cold compress to the wrist and base of the hand can relieve symptoms.

🐇 Natural Supplements

▶ High-Dose B Vitamins

The most common form of B6, pyridoxine, can be effective but possibly toxic in high doses above 100 mg. Another form of B6, which is found in the human body and called pyridoxal-5-phosphate, is not toxic, even with doses as high as 500 mg a day. However, studies have shown that a mixture of the B vitamins works better. A B complex should include B6 in the form of pyridoxal-5-phosphate, thiamine (B1) in the form of riboflavin-5-phosphate, niacinamide, biotin, folate, and methylcobalamin (B12). Each of these B vitamins plays a role in nerve health and function. B-Complex Plus, made by Pure Encapsulations, is a well-designed B complex product.

> ➡ **What to do:** Take one capsule of B-Complex Plus, three times a day until well, then one capsule, twice a day.

▶ Fish Oil

Omega-3 oils in fish reduce inflammation through a number of mechanisms that help with carpal tunnel syndrome. Liquid Fish

Oil, made by Carlson, comes in an orange or lemon flavor and is an easy way to get a therapeutic dose.

➡ **What to do:** Take two teaspoons of the Carlson liquid fish oil, three times a day.

▶ Carnitine

Also called L-carnitine, it plays a role in nerve function and repair. A number of studies have shown that it improves nerve healing after damage by compression or other injuries.

➡ **What to do:** Take 500 to 1,500 mg, two to three times a day, 30 minutes before meals.

▶ R-Lipoic acid

A potent antioxidant produced by every cell in the body, it promotes nerve healing.

➡ **What to do:** Take 300 mg, three times a day with meals.

▶ Curcumin and Quercetin

Working together, these two natural substances have been shown to significantly protect nerves, promote healing from nerve injury, and prevent prolonged nerve pain from developing. It's important to take products that are well absorbed, such as CurcumaSorb, made by Pure Encapsulations, and Quercenase, made by Thorne Research. Both contain 250 mg per capsule.

➡ **What to do:** Take two capsules each of CurcumaSorb and Quercenase, three times a day with meals.

▶ Green Tea Extract (EGCG)

Studies have shown that EGCG, a therapeutic component in green and white tea, reduces the damage caused by crushing a nerve. It also promotes repair and healing of damaged nerves. In supplements, EGCG usually comes from green tea.

What to do: Take 100 mg, twice a day with meals. Or, drink two cups of strong white tea, twice a day.

Fibromyalgia

In the United States, fibromyalgia—once called fibrositis—is the most common cause of widespread chronic pain, meaning it affects many parts of the body. It has been described as a deep pain in muscles and ligaments, with stabbing, shooting, and throbbing sensations, as well as numbness, tingling, and burning. Pain and stiffness are often worse in the morning, when the weather is cold or humid, after unusual amounts of physical activity or inactivity, and when an individual is under more stress than usual. Depression is common and may precede the onset of the diffuse muscle pains.

It's estimated that up to 4 percent of the population suffers from fibromyalgia, and most are women. African American women are affected more than Caucasians. Sleep disturbances, debilitating fatigue, mental fog, and sensitivity to touch, sound, and light are other common signs. Even after a long sleep, people with fibromyalgia typically don't feel refreshed. Most consider fibromyalgia a life-long disorder.

POSSIBLE SYMPTOMS

In addition to widespread pain, exhaustion, mental fog, extreme sensitivity to touch, and sleep problems, people suffering from fibromyalgia may also experience one or more of these symptoms:

- Anxiety
- Depression
- Weight gain
- Dry eyes
- Dry mouth
- Allergies and chemical sensitivities
- Heart palpitations
- Bladder problems
- Pain in the chest or hips

Conventional Treatment

From a conventional medical perspective, fibromyalgia is considered to be a genetic disorder that is triggered by a stressful event, which could be a traumatic life incident, an injury, or an illness, such as an infection or autoimmune disease. The condition affects the central nervous system and amplifies pain and other sensations that are not usually painful. As an example, a massage could be excruciatingly painful.

Conventional medical treatment does not offer a cure but aims to reduce the severity of symptoms with various medications. These include anti-depressants, pain relievers, and insomnia drugs, all having significant side effects. Lifestyle changes, including improvements in diet, stress reduction, and physical activity can help to bring relief.

👍 My Recommendations

There is considerable evidence that excitotoxicity and inflammation play major roles in this condition. This interaction between inflammation and excitotoxicity is called immunoexcitotoxicity, a mechanism described in more detail in the "Excitotoxins" chapter. Immunoexcitotoxicity is what causes the pain pathways in the brain and spinal cord to become amplified and overactive. As a result, even normal sensations can cause pain, other discomfort, and more serious neurological signs and symptoms.

Many things can trigger immunoexcitotoxicity, such as infections, trauma, stress, autoimmune diseases, and exposure to toxic metals, pesticides, and herbicides. Glutamate, as found in MSG in many processed foods, and aspartic acid in aspartame, the artificial sugar substitute, are major excitotoxins.

While dietary excitotoxins may not be the sole cause of fibromyalgia in genetically susceptible people, they definitely worsen symptoms. In one study, researchers examined four women with severe fibromyalgia who did not respond to any treatments for up to 17 years. They found that removing all excitotoxins and aspartame from their diets resulted in dramatic improvements in all the women. A later, carefully conducted study, involving 57 fibromyalgia patients, also found that removing excitotoxins and aspartame from the diets resulted in 84 percent experiencing significant improvements, with more than 30 percent of their symptoms disappearing. In another test among women who did improve, researchers gave them placebos or MSG to see if their symptoms would return. Those getting the MSG, but not the placebo, experienced a significant worsening of their symptoms.

A great many foods contain excitotoxins, often under disguised names, such as hydrolyzed vegetable protein, soy protein extract and isolate, soy sauce, natural flavoring, autolyzed yeast, carrageenan, stock, and vegetable powder—just to name a few. The only real way to avoid excitotoxins is to eat only organically grown vegetables and fruits and make vegetables and some fruits your main meal. Some foods naturally contain high levels of glutamate, such as tomatoes (especially when pureed or made into a sauce), mushrooms, cheeses, meats, nuts (especially peanuts), chickpeas, sweet peas, and soy foods and sauces. These should be avoided. Both white and red sauces often contain high levels of glutamate, as do many salad dressings.

These are some other important things to keep in mind:

- Exercise should be done in moderation and with sufficient warm up. Intense exercise can worsen symptoms.

- Obesity increases risk as fat cells release inflammatory substances. Losing fat, especially abdominal fat, greatly reduces the inflammation.

- Drink plenty of purified water.

- Avoid all fluoride, not only in water but also in dental treatments, toothpaste, and mouthwash.

- Mercury can significantly trigger immunoexcitotoxicity. Major sources include vaccines (such as flu shots), dental amalgam fillings, seafood (especially shark, swordfish, tile fish, and grouper), and industrial facilities that burn coal or make brick.

- Exposure to lead can also worsen immunoexcitotoxicity.

It is also important to maintain healthy probiotics—beneficial bacteria in the gut. Low concentrations of colon probiotics can result in chronic inflammation. In probiotic supplements, look for a variety of beneficial bacteria. I recommend buying a refrigerated product with a guarantee of its potency.

In addition, there is some evidence that those affected by fibromyalgia suffer from impaired energy production due to abnormalities in mitochondria, the energy-generating components of all cells, and low levels of coenzyme Q10. Called CoQ10 for short, this is a vital nutrient required by the mitochondria in the production of energy. In food, organ meats are the richest sources, yet these are not part of our usual diet.

Natural Supplements

The most important supplements are those that reduce inflammation or reduce excitotoxicity, and many do both.

▶ Magnesium Malate

Magnesium is a major inhibitor of inflammation. It also enhances energy production, improves blood flow in microvessels, inhibits excitotoxicity, prevents blood clots, and is essential for normal immune function.

➡ **What to do:** Take a slow-release form of magnesium malate called Magnesium w/SRT, made by Jigsaw Health. I favor this product as it maintains a constant magnesium level in tissues, is less likely to cause diarrhea from high doses, and enhances energy. For severe cases, take two caplets, three times a day with meals. For less severe cases, two caplets taken twice a day with meals should be sufficient.

▶ Apigenin

This is a natural flavonoid found in celery and parsley. It also comes as a purified supplement. A number of studies have shown that it quiets the cells that generate the inflammatory and excitotoxic compounds.

➡ **What to do:** Take two capsules (100 mg), three times a day of Apigenin, made by Swanson. For severe cases, the dose can be increased to four capsules (200 mg), three times a day.

▶ Luteolin

A flavonoid found in celery and artichoke luteolin reduces immunoexcitotoxicity and inflammation, enhances memory, and protects the brain and central nervous system. And, it is a powerful antioxidant. One study found that combining apigenin and luteolin significantly cleared brain fog associated with fibromyalgia, food allergies, and gluten sensitivity. Luteolin Complex, made by Swanson, is a good product.

➡ **What to do:** Take one capsule (100 mg), three times a day with meals. For severe cases, increase the dose to three capsules, three times a day with meals.

▶ Multivitamin/Mineral

The best product includes ample B vitamins, as these not only enhance energy production but also suppress excitotoxicity. I prefer a multivitamin without iron, such as Extend Core, made by Vitamin Research Products. For those with a diagnosed iron deficiency, an iron supplement can be taken separately.

➡ **What to do:** Take one capsule of Extend Core, three times a day with meals, or follow directions for the product of your choice.

▶ DHA

Short for docosahexaenoic acid, DHA is a component of omega-3 oils found in fish. It is one of the most abundant fats in the brain and is a building block of neuron membranes and junctions between nerve cells, called synapses. It inhibits excitotoxicity, reduces inflammation, and plays a major role in repairing damaged cells. DHA is also found in certain types of algae.

➡ **What to do:** Take 1,000 to 2,000 mg a day of DHA, from fish oil or algae.

▶ Coenzyme Q10 (CoQ10)

Several studies have shown lower CoQ10 levels in those with fibromyalgia. Supplementing with CoQ10 has had mixed results, most likely because of poor absorption of some brands. Mixing CoQ10 with oil, such as coconut oil or extra virgin olive oil, improves absorption. Some products are formulated with an oil to improve absorption. A "nanosized" form of CoQ10 also improves absorption.

➡ **What to do:** Higher doses appear to be more effective, and may be as high as 500 to 600 mg, three times a day with meals.

▶ Mixed Tocopherols and Tocotrienols

In nature, vitamin E is a family of nutrients composed of four compounds called tocopherols, and four compounds called tocotrienols. Together, they have strong antioxidant and anti-inflammatory effects, and protect the brain and nervous system.

➡ **What to do:** Take 400 IU of mixed tocopherols and 50 mg of mixed tocotrienols, twice a day with meals.

▶ Buffered Vitamin C

Although vitamin C is known to be an antioxidant, it does much more. It regulates neurotransmitters, reduces inflammation, enhances immunity, stimulates cellular energy production, and has anticancer, antiviral, and antibacterial effects. Lypo-Spheric Vitamin C, made by LivOn Labs, is a highly absorbable, buffered form that is non-acidic and easy on the stomach. It comes in packets of gel that can be mixed with water or other liquids. When taken with food, vitamin C increases absorption of iron and can lead to iron overload, which is harmful to the brain.

High doses of ordinary vitamin C supplements, which are usually acidic, can cause digestive upset.

➡ **What to do:** Take 1 packet (1,000 mg) of Lypo-Spheric Vitamin C, three times a day between meals.

▶ Curcumin

Curcumin is a flavonoid found in higher concentrations in the curry spice turmeric. Many studies have found it to be a very powerful compound for protecting the brain. It reduces inflammation in the muscles, connective tissues, and brain. Studies using massive doses found it to have a very high margin of safety. When dissolved in an oil, such as coconut or extra virgin olive oil, it is well absorbed and enters the brain very easily from the blood.

➡ **What to do:** Take 250 to 500 mg, three times a day, with meals. Use a highly absorbable form such as CurcumaSorb, made by Pure Encapsulations. Or, mix the powder contents of a capsule with a tablespoon of coconut or extra virgin olive oil. This can be messy.

▶ Quercetin

This is a flavonoid found in plants, such as tea, onions, parsley, and apples. It has powerful antioxidant and anti-inflammatory effects and is even more effective when taken with curcumin.

➡ **What to do:** Take 250 to 500 mg, three times a day, of a form that is well absorbed, such as Quercenase, made by Thorne Research.

▶ Hyperbaric Oxygen Therapy (HBOT)

Hyperbaric oxygen therapy, with 100 percent oxygen at elevated atmospheric pressures, holds much promise in reversing fibromyalgia symptoms. One well done study found that even after one treatment, pain was significantly reduced and the pain threshold was elevated, meaning tender spots became much less sensitive. Testing after 15 treatments demonstrated even greater effectiveness.

Gout

A form of arthritis, gout affects more than 3 million Americans. Although men are most prone to the disease, especially if it runs in their family, women become more susceptible after menopause. People with kidney disease are also at higher risk.

Symptoms most often begin in the big toe but can affect any joint, and include sudden, severe incidents of pain, swelling, stiffness, tenderness, and redness. The disease is a result of elevated levels of uric acid, a normal waste product of the human body, which leads to deposits of sharp-edged crystals in joints. Most often, the kidneys are not able to eliminate uric acid as they should, or excess levels may be produced.

> **TRIGGERS OF GOUT ATTACKS**
>
> Certain foods, which are high in a naturally occurring substance called purines, and drugs can trigger gout attacks because they raise levels of uric acid. These include:
>
> - Red meat, shellfish, anchovies, organ meats, and mushrooms
> - Alcoholic drinks, especially beer, and hard liquor, to a lesser extent
> - Beverages and foods high in fructose
> - Low-dose aspirin
> - Some diuretic medications
> - Immunosuppressant drugs taken in connection with organ transplants

Conventional Treatment

Colchicine is a drug used to prevent and treat gout attacks, but its side effects include nausea, vomiting, and diarrhea. Over-the-counter anti-inflammatory drugs are also used for pain relief. Other medications may be prescribed to reduce levels of uric acid, either by blocking its production or helping the kidneys to remove it, but these do not relieve symptoms during an attack.

My Recommendations

Abstaining from foods rich in purines is a basic strategy for preventing gout attacks. Purines are components of virtually all foods, but some, such as meats and seafood, contain higher amounts. Although some vegetables also contain higher levels of purines—including asparagus, cauliflower, green peas, spinach, mushrooms, and dried beans and lentils—these do not appear to cause problems. However, gout sufferers typically eat fewer vegetables and drink more sweetened beverages than those without gout. Coffee lowers levels of uric acid.

Natural Supplements

A common gout drug, Allopurinol, lowers uric acid levels by blocking the enzyme xanthine oxidase. A number of plant chemicals, in the class of nutrients called flavonoids, are also powerful inhibitors of the same enzyme but are much safer than the prescription drug. Extracts that inhibit the enzyme include quercetin, luteolin, baicalein, and green tea extract. Some of the other supplements below reduce gout pain by a different mechanism and all work in multiple ways. These nutrients are found in many commonly eaten fruits and vegetables.

▶ Luteolin

Luteolin is a flavonoid found in high concentrations in celery and artichoke. As well as inhibiting the enzyme used in making uric acid, it reduces inflammation and calms an overactive immune system.

➡ **What to do:** Take 100 mg, three times a day with meals.

▶ Quercetin

In addition to suppressing the xanthine oxidase enzyme, quercetin calms immune reactions and inflammation that occurs with gout and other joint conditions. Use a product that is well absorbed such as Quercenase, made by Thorne Research, which contains 250 mg per capsule.

➡ **What to do:** Take 500 to 1,000 mg of Quercenase, three times a day with meals. For good absorption of other brands, open capsules, mix the powder with coconut oil, and take the mixture.

▶ Baicalein

This is a compound found in the skullcap plant. It has powerful anti-inflammatory effects and strongly suppresses the xanthine oxidase enzyme. You can buy pure baicalein, which comes in a jar with a measuring spoon.

> ➧ **What to do:** Mix a half of one measuring spoon of powder in a tablespoon of extra virgin olive oil and take this twice a day with meals.

▶ Green Tea Extract (EGCG)

One of the components of green tea, EGCG is an extract that inhibits the xanthine oxidase enzyme and thus lowers uric acid levels. A standardized extract, called Teavigo, is found in several brands of supplements.

> ➧ **What to do:** Take 100 mg, three times a day with meals.

▶ Grape Seed Extract

Although it is not a strong inhibitor of the uric-acid producing enzyme, grape seed extract works in multiple ways to lower blood levels of uric acid, and it lowers inflammation and harmful immune activation. It is dose-dependent, meaning the more you use it, the better the results. To reduce the number of capsules you have to take, I recommend Grape Seed Extract, made by Bestvite, which contains 500 mg per capsule.

> ➧ **What to do:** Take 500 mg, two to three times a day with meals.

▶ Hesperidin

A flavonoid found in high concentrations in oranges, hesperidin has been extensively studied and found to effectively reduce inflammation and depression—especially depression with anxiety. It does not inhibit the xanthine oxidase enzyme.

➡ **What to do:** Take 500 to 1,000 mg, three times a day with meals.

▶ **Pycnogenol**

An extract of French maritime pine bark, Pycnogenol is a natural anti-inflammatory and reduces gout pain by reducing inflammation of joints. It does not inhibit the xanthine oxidase enzyme.

➡ **What to do:** Take 100 mg, three times a day with meals.

Headaches and Migraines

Headaches all have one thing in common—pain—but there are different types. The most common is a tension headache, with tight muscles in the neck, shoulders, or jaw. Tension headaches are characterized by a feeling that a tight band is around the head. Migraines, the second most common, manifest with more severe pain and have additional symptoms, such as feeling nauseous or having changes in vision. Newer studies suggest that in many cases, these distinctions are artificial, that is, most headaches have features of both migraines and tension headaches. The common link is inflammation and excitotoxicity, described in more detail in chapter 2.

Other types of headaches may be associated with women's menstrual cycles, sinus infections, a cold, flu, or fever. Less often, a headache may be a sign of something more serious, such as an infection or swelling in the brain, very high blood pressure, a brain tumor, or rupture of brain blood vessels. (Ironically, in many cases of brain tumors, there is no headache.) Another common cause of headache is hypoglycemia—a sudden drop in blood sugar. Hypoglycemic headaches are usually very severe and unrelenting, sometimes lasting for many hours, and are very resistant to treatment with the usual painkillers.

Headaches that signify serious disorders are preceded or followed by neurological symptoms, such as weakness in a limb, numbness in a limb, or a loss of speech. When a gradual loss of consciousness accompanies a headache, one should seek emergency care immediately.

Conventional Treatment

Beyond taking a pain reliever, which is not advised as a longer-term approach, conventional treatment for tension and migraine headaches includes staying hydrated by drinking water, resting in a quiet room that is dark or has low light, applying a cool compress to the head, and relaxing in whatever way works for you.

For other types of headaches, the underlying condition needs to be treated or allowed to heal. To check for serious underlying medical problems, physicians might use blood tests, an MRI or CT scan, special x-rays of the brain, or a lumbar puncture to collect spinal fluid, which is then analyzed in a lab.

MIGRAINE SYMPTOMS

There are several forms of migraine headaches, including a type in which there is no headache but rather visual aura—flashing lights in one's visual field, much like a squiggly neon sign. Migraines tend to occur on one side of the head and may be preceded by visual aura, difficulty thinking, confusion, or disorientation. They can occur at any age and may start for the first time at middle age. Migraines that appear later in life and have visual phenomena are strongly connected to a risk of stroke. A common link in both is that there is usually a significant magnesium deficiency.

Migraine symptoms often include:

- Nausea
- Vomiting
- Vision changes
- Diarrhea
- Sensitivity to light or sound
- A pale face
- Dizziness
- Ringing in the ears
- Tenderness on the scalp
- A pulsing pain

👍 My Recommendations

Diet can play a major role in preventing or aggravating migraines or tension headaches. A high-sugar diet plays a major role in both types of headaches because sugar depletes the body's magnesium, can precipitate severe drops in blood sugar, and increases inflammation. Sugar should be eliminated from the diet.

Many medications, both prescription and over-the-counter, severely deplete the body's magnesium. Magnesium is important in preventing headaches because it reduces inflammation, especially within blood vessels, reduces excitotoxicity, and relaxes muscles in the neck.

A number of foods can precipitate migraine headaches. These include seafood, chocolate, excessive caffeine, aged cheeses, alcohol, MSG, and other food additives with glutamate (listed in chapter 2), peanuts, dried fruits, cultured dairy products, soy foods, soy beverages, soy-based food ingredients, and foods and drinks sweetened with the zero-calorie sweetener aspartame. It's essential to avoid these.

In contrast, vegetables contain a number of flavonoids that reduce inflammation and block excitotoxicity. And, they are an excellent source of magnesium. Two vegetables should be avoided as they are extremely high in nitric oxide—spinach and beets. Supplements that specifically increase nitric oxide should also be avoided.

Other ways to prevent migraines and headaches include biofeedback, regular exercise, and massage therapy. Stress relief is equally important. Getting enough sleep is a starting point, along with managing one's schedule and obligations, and setting aside time for enjoyable activities.

🐰 Natural Supplements

▶ Magnesium

Magnesium reduces inflammation inside the blood vessels in the brain and in those feeding the scalp, which are most involved in migraines and possibly tension headaches. The malate or citrate forms are best, in a slow-release form, such as Magnesium w/SRT, made by Jigsaw Health. It is easy on the gut and provides the brain with a continuous source of magnesium.

➡ **What to do:** Take two 250 mg capsules, three times a day. For severe attacks, I recommend a solution of magnesium citrate and/or malate powder. Empty the contents of six or seven capsules (not in a slow-release form) in a glass of water and drink the entire mixture. This will raise your magnesium level rapidly and can often terminate an attack.

▶ Hesperidin

Found in high concentrations in oranges, hesperidin reduces pain and calms nerves, which reduces stress. I have found it to be a useful sleep aid as well.

➡ **What to do:** Take 500 to 1,000 mg, one to three times a day, as needed.

▶ Feverfew

Feverfew, a plant, is one of the oldest remedies for migraines. It contains a compound called parthenolide, which appears to be the active ingredient. In most cases, the longer the supplement is taken, the more effective it becomes in preventing migraines.

➡ **What to do:** Take 50 to 100 mg a day.

▶ Riboflavin-5-phosphate (R-5-P)

This is a special form of riboflavin, vitamin B2. It is the form found naturally in the human body and when taken in supplements, is especially beneficial. High doses have been shown to reduce the frequency and intensity of migraines. A good high-dose product is R-5-P, made by Swanson Health Products, which contains 50 mg per capsule.

➧ **What to do:** Take 50 to 100 mg, twice a day with or without meals.

▶ R-Lipoic Acid

Several studies have shown a reduction in frequency and severity of migraine headaches with regular use of R-lipoic acid. R-lipoic acid can significantly lower blood sugar, and individuals with significant reactive hypoglycemia may get worse using this supplement. In that case it should be avoided.

➧ **What to do:** Take 100 mg, three times a day with meals. Beware: if taken without food, it can lower blood sugar too severely.

▶ Hyperbaric Oxygen Therapy (HBOT)

Some studies have shown that HBOT improves headaches, especially those classed as migraines or other types of vascular headaches. HBOT treatments would be reserved for headaches that are unresponsive to less expensive types of treatment.

Joint Pain (Acute)

Acute joint pain is most often the result of a sprain or strain, or overuse during exercise, sports, work, or other activity. Joint pain from overuse usually subsides within a few days. If in doubt, see a doctor, as untreated injuries can lead to infections or permanent damage. Most acute injuries involve either torn or strained ligaments, torn joint cartilage, or tendon injuries. In more serious cases, all of these body parts may be injured.

With any injury, one of the responses by the body is to initiate an inflammatory response at the site. This causes pain, swelling, and redness. While we do not like this, it is part of the healing process. Our goal should be to prevent excess inflammation, while at the same time stimulating healing of the injury.

Conventional Treatment

For an injury, x-rays and a physical exam are standard. For soft tissue injuries, such as an ankle sprain, first aid usually includes RICE: rest, to prevent aggravation of the injured area; ice every few hours; compression with a bandage or tape to reduce swelling; and elevation, also to reduce swelling. Treatment for other joint injuries depends upon the diagnosis.

My Recommendations

Acute joint pain due to injures requires immobilization using elastic bandages or special supports, most available for purchase from pharmacies. It is important to apply a cold compress immediately to acute joint injuries.

> **CHRONIC JOINT PAIN**
>
> Rheumatoid arthritis, osteoarthritis, and gout are common causes of chronic joint pain. Rheumatoid arthritis is an autoimmune disorder with severe destructive inflammation occurring in numerous joints. Osteoarthritis has been considered a wear-and-tear disorder but is now recognized as also being inflammatory, with a much lower level of inflammation than rheumatoid arthritis. Gout is triggered by excessive levels of uric acid, as covered above in the "Gout" section. For more on osteoarthritis and rheumatoid arthritis, see the relevant sections in chapter 14, "Chronic Conditions.". Repetitive, focused activities, such as tennis or golf, are also common causes for chronic joint pain, and weak muscles or tendons can contribute to pain.

The cold reduces swelling, pain, and redness (inflammation) and helps prevent hemorrhaging within the joint. After 12 to 24 hours, a warm compress can then be applied, which will improve blood flow to the area, reduce pain, and improve mobility. Hot compresses should be avoided.

Natural Supplements

▶ MSM (Methylsulfonylmethane)

There are two ways MSM can be used—orally or topically in a cream. For acute joint injuries, I prefer a topical cream. MSM has some anti-inflammatory effects and reduces swelling of the injured joint. Various MSM creams are available or you can make your own.

➡ **What to do:** Use an MSM cream or lotion or, to make your own, mix about 1 ounce of an MSM powder with 4 ounces of a base cream, such as Derma e Vitamin E Intensive Therapy Body Lotion. Rub the MSM lotion on the injured area three times a day until healed.

▶ **Curcumin**

One of the impressive properties of curcumin is that it stimulates healing of injured tissues, as well as reduces excessive inflammation. Use a well-absorbed form such as CurcumaSorb, made by Pure Encapsulations.

➡ **What to do:** Take 500 mg, three times a day with meals.

▶ **Quercetin**

Like curcumin, quercetin reduces inflammation and pain and speeds healing, but it works in a slightly different way, so the two are complementary. A well-absorbed form is Quercenase, made by Thorne Research.

➡ **What to do:** Take 250 mg, three times a day with meals.

▶ **Wobenzym N**

This is an enzyme, often used by athletes for treating injuries. It helps healing of joints, muscles, and other soft tissues. In supplements, it is available in multiple brands of products.

➡ **What to do:** Take three tablets on an empty stomach, preferably at least three hours before a meal.

▶ **Vitamin C**

Vitamin C plays a major role in strengthening and healing tendons, ligaments, and other soft tissues that support joints. Low levels of vitamin C weaken tendons and ligaments, making joints less resilient to stress and more susceptible to injury. Use a form that is well-absorbed; even a high dose will not be fully effective. Lypo-Spheric Vitamin C, made by LivOn Labs, is an absorbable form that is not acidic and is well tolerated. It comes in packets of gel which is mixed with water or juice. Each packet contains 1,000 mg of vitamin C.

➡ **What to do:** Take two packets (2,000 mg) of Lypo-Spheric Vitamin C, three times a day.

▶ Hyperbaric Oxygen Therapy (HBOT)

Some studies have shown improvement in joint pain with HBOT. This is not surprising, since HBOT has been shown to reduce inflammation, and inflammation plays a significant role in joint pain.

—— Kidney Stones ——

It's estimated that one in twenty people will have kidney stones at sometime in life. The degree of discomfort can vary dramatically, from a minimal amount to excruciating pain and other symptoms. In many cases, kidney stones run in families, and are more likely to form among people who have gout.

The stones are made of salts and minerals, most often calcium oxalate, and can be as small as a grain of sand or as big as a golf ball. They form in the kid-

> **SYMPTOMS OF KIDNEY STONES**
>
> When kidney stones move out of the kidney and start to pass through the urinary tract, symptoms may include:
> - Severe pain in the back, side, abdomen, groin, or genitals
> - Pink or red urine
> - Nausea
> - Vomiting
> - Painful urination

neys and don't cause pain as long as they stay there. Symptoms usually begin as a stone moves out and starts to pass through the urinary tract, which includes tubes that connect the kidney to the bladder (called ureters), the bladder itself, and the urethra, the tube that carries urine out of the body. Kidney stone pain is classed as one of the worst a person can endure.

☜ Conventional Treatment

Kidney stones are diagnosed with ultrasound or CT scans. Some are eliminated on their own with little discomfort, or with some pain medication. Stones that are too big to pass may be broken up with medication or shock waves, called extracorporeal shock wave lithotripsy, or ESWL. In other cases, a stent may be inserted into the urinary tract to help eliminate stones. The use of surgery is very rare.

👍 My Recommendations

Urine that is darker in color and low in volume indicates insufficient fluids, and this increases risk for kidney stones. (However, B vitamins, especially riboflavin, give the urine a bright yellow color, even in a well-hydrated person.) Drinking plenty of water helps prevent stones from forming and aids in their elimination.

The most common form of kidney stone is made of calcium oxalate. Plant foods naturally contain oxalate, to varying degrees. Avoiding foods high in oxalate, such as chocolate, spinach, rhubarb, beets, potato chips, French fries, nuts, and nut butters, can reduce risk of developing kidney stones. Other, less common stones may be associated with urinary tract infections. These may be silent and can get quite large. Uric acid stones, linked to gout, are another type. They usually result from drinking insufficient fluids and eating a high protein diet.

There has been a belief that vitamin C can increase the risk of calcium oxalate stones. But according to numerous studies of individuals taking massive doses of vitamin C, this is not the case. Vitamin C does not cause kidney stones.

The best way to prevent the most common, calcium oxalate stones, is to drink a small glass of organic orange juice at least once a day. Magnesium and acidic substances with which it is combined in some supplements, such as citrate or malate, also prevent kidney stones.

Natural Supplements

▶ Magnesium Citrate or Malate

Magnesium is a powerful relaxant for smooth muscle, the type of muscle that lines the ureters and urethra. It also reduces inflammation and blocks the formation of kidney stones. In some supplements, magnesium is bound with either malate or citrate, substances that also inhibit stone formation. Magnesium can also end a kidney stone attack, relieving the excruciating pain when the stone irritates the ureter and triggers an intense spasm.

➡ **What to do:** For acute kidney stone pain, mix 8 ounces of filtered water and 1 scoop (250 mg) of Magnesium Powder (contains citrate), made by Pure Encapsulations, and drink it quickly. For prevention of stones, use a slow-release form of magnesium malate called Magnesium w/SRT, made by Jigsaw Health. Take two caplets, two or three times a day, with meals.

CHAPTER 9

Digestion

Celiac Disease and Gluten

Many people avoid gluten because they feel better on such a diet or believe it is a healthier way to eat, but those with celiac disease must avoid it or face significant health risks. Celiac disease is an autoimmune disorder caused by a reaction to gluten, found naturally in most grains, which damages the inner lining of the small intestine. Most of the damage is to the villi, tiny finger-like projections that are responsible for most of the food absorption in the intestines. Damage to these villi can interfere with nutrients being properly absorbed and may lead to other health conditions.

Although the cause of celiac disease is unknown, there may be a genetic predisposition. It may appear at any age. Many cases are not diagnosed for decades, leading to a lifetime of misery and illness. Often, the disorder begins in childhood and the symptoms are dismissed as growing pains, bad behavior, and malingering.

The resulting nutritional deficiencies are frequently overlooked and can lead to serious disorders. Iron deficiency anemia, for example, is common. In adults, peripheral neuropathies are frequent, often misdiagnosed as numbness and pain of unknown cause. Gluten intolerance is one of the most common causes for cerebellar ataxia, which manifests as loss of the sense of balance and coordination. Cancer and unexplained female infertility are other possible consequences. The longer the condition goes undiagnosed, the more likely it is that a major complication will develop.

In about half of all cases, celiac disease runs in families. It is diagnosed with a blood test for certain antibodies, and intestinal and skin biopsies may also be done. People with celiac disease may also suffer from other autoimmune conditions, such as rheumatoid arthritis, type 1 diabetes, multiple sclerosis, autoimmune hepatitis, dilated cardiomyopathy, dermatitis herpetiformis (also called Duhring's disease), migraines, seizures, and intestinal cancers.

SYMPTOMS OF CELIAC DISEASE

These are some symptoms that may be present with untreated celiac disease, although they may also be signs of other disorders:

- Stomach pain or bloating
- Chronic constipation or diarrhea
- Gas
- Severe weight loss
- Nausea or vomiting
- Mood problems or irritability
- In children, delayed puberty
- Anemia
- Infertility
- Fatigue
- Mouth sores
- Skin rash and itching
- Pain in the joints or bones
- Headaches
- Tingling or numbness in the hands and feet
- Weakness and/or muscle atrophy in the legs
- Infertility

Gluten intolerance is much more common than full-blown celiac disease and can be much more difficult to diagnose. One expert in gluten-related disease told me that everyone is sensitive to gluten if eating high enough concentrations. Modern wheat products have much higher gluten levels than previous wheat crops, and gluten is added to a great many processed foods. In some people, even a very small amount of gluten can precipitate a health crisis.

Screening for gluten sensitivity can be done with the tTG-IgA (tissue transglutaminase IgA antibody) test, which is 98 percent accurate in patients with celiac disease. Other highly accurate tests include the IgA-endomysial antibody test and the gliadin antibody test.

Conventional Treatment

Avoiding gluten is the only treatment for celiac disease since even small amounts can cause damage. Although grains are the source of gluten in nature, it may also be found as a food additive in many packaged foods and other products, including medications, nutritional and herbal products, lipsticks and other cosmetics, skin and hair care products, toothpastes and mouthwashes, and in glue on stamps and envelopes. However, more and more foods and other products are now being manufactured without gluten, and these are labeled "gluten- free."

My Recommendations

At present, there is no way around avoiding foods containing gluten. Corn naturally contains no gluten but make sure it is not GMO corn, which may contain allergens. All foods with wheat, rye, barley, and other sources of gluten should be eliminated from the diet. However, gluten-free packaged or baked foods can be problematic in another way. Most are made from rice, which is high in starch, and very rapidly converts to blood sugar. This rapid conversion can trigger a condition called reactive hypoglycemia, which is dangerously low blood sugar within four hours after eating. This can be a major problem in those already suffering from reactive hypoglycemia or neurological problems associated with gluten sensitivity.

For anyone who is sensitive to gluten or has celiac disease, most carbohydrate needs can be met by eating a high-vegetable diet, legumes, and berries. There are some digestive enzyme products that claim to reduce risk by breaking down gluten into a non-allergenic molecular size, but so far, this has not been proven. Digestive enzyme supplements may be helpful but are not, as yet, an alternative to avoiding gluten. It would be helpful if manufacturers of processed foods stopped adding extra gluten to their products. As it is, it's vital to check ingredient lists of all prepared or packaged foods to see if they contain gluten.

Natural Supplements

One of the goals for supplementation is to make sure the individual gets all of the vitamins and minerals that are not absorbed as a result of celiac disease. Once gluten is completely eliminated, absorption may return to normal. Reducing intestinal inflammation will aid in recovery. It has been noted that even when gluten has been eliminated from the diet, cancer risk is still elevated and some neurological conditions do not improve. This may be because of continuing inflammation resulting from gluten and gliadin components of grain that have been trapped in the walls of the intestine or other tissues, thus allowing a continued immune attack. All supplements should be gluten-free.

▶ Multivitamins and Minerals

A multivitamin and mineral supplement plus extra vitamin C and E are basic, essential nutrients. The multivitamin should contain high doses of B vitamins, vitamin A as mixed carotenoids or beta-carotene, and all of the minerals and trace elements. The multivitamin should not contain iron. If an iron deficiency has been diagnosed, a separate iron supplement can be taken, as and when needed. Vitamin C should be buffered to avoid digestive upset and should generally be taken between meals, as it increases absorption of iron from food and can lead to an iron overload. Vitamin E should contain a family of vitamin E nutrients, called mixed tocopherols, to mimic nature. The specific products I mention below fit these criteria.

➡ **What to do:** For a multivitamin, take Extend Core, made by Vitamin Research Products, one capsule, three times a day with meals. Take vitamin E as mixed tocopherols, 400 IU a day. For vitamin C, take Lypo-Spheric Vitamin C, made by LivOn Labs, which comes in packets of gel that can be mixed with water or juice. Take one packet (1,000 mg) three times a day between meals. However, if iron deficiency is a problem, take vitamin C with meals, for increased absorption of iron from food.

▶ Apigenin

This is a natural flavonoid found in celery and parsley. A number of studies have shown that it quiets inflammation and harmful immune reactions.

➡ **What to do:** Take 100 mg (two capsules), three times a day, of Swanson's Apigenin. In severe cases, the dose can be increased to four capsules, three times a day.

▶ Luteolin

A flavonoid found in celery and artichokes luteolin reduces harmful immune reactions and inflammation, enhances memory, and protects the brain and central nervous system. And, it is a powerful antioxidant. One study found that combining apigenin and luteolin significantly cleared brain fog associated with gluten sensitivity, food allergies, and fibromyalgia. Luteolin Complex, made by Swanson, is a good product.

➡ **What to do:** Take one capsule (100 mg), three times a day with meals. For severe cases, increase the dose to three capsules, three times a day with meals.

▶ DHA

Short for docosahexaenoic acid, DHA is a component of omega-3 oils found in fish. It is one of the most abundant fats in the brain and is a building block of neuron membranes and junctions between nerve cells, called synapses. It inhibits excitotoxicity, reduces inflammation, and plays a major role in repairing damaged cells. DHA is also found in certain types of algae.

➡ **What to do:** Take 1,000 to 2,000 mg a day of DHA, from fish oil or algae.

Constipation

Constipation is defined by the National Institute of Diabetes and Digestive and Kidney Diseases as having three or less bowel movements per week. That agency also considers that it is not necessary to have a bowel movement daily, but many holistic and integrative practitioners disagree. It is my opinion that, at any age, a person should have at least one bowel movement a day.

When constipation occurs, the muscles and nerves related to elimination may not be functioning optimally—the longer the constipation problem, the more likely the neural control of the bowel will be functioning abnormally. Damage to these nerves is common with aging. Although the cause is sometimes unknown, dietary habits can contribute by providing insufficient fiber and moisture. For this or possibly other reasons, food moves through the digestive tract too slowly, creating an internal traffic jam. Constipation can also be a side effect of medications.

Chronic constipation can lead to abnormal growth of colon bacteria, a condition called dysbiosis. This can lead to harmful bacteria entering the small intestine, and even the stomach, which can result in a number of digestive problems such as bloating, abdominal cramping, and heartburn.

One of the primary functions of the colon (the large bowel) is re-absorption of water as protection from dehydration. Normally, the colon re-absorbs about a quart of water a day. Older people often suffer from mild to moderate degrees of dehydration, which increases the absorption of water from the bowel, causing the stool to become hard and dry.

> **SYMPTOMS OF CONSTIPATION**
>
> In addition to having too few bowel movements, these are some other symptoms:
> - Stools that are hard, dry, and difficult to pass
> - Straining to have a bowel movement
> - Feeling that there is a blockage preventing elimination
> - Having fewer bowel movements than usual

Conventional Treatment

Although they are a common remedy, laxatives can become a crutch and often make things worse. This is especially true of laxatives that stimulate colon muscle contraction, as they can damage the controlling nerves. Basic dietary advice for regularity includes eating more high-fiber plant foods, especially vegetables, drinking plenty of liquids, getting regular exercise, and allowing time to have a bowel movement.

Certain medical conditions can also cause or contribute to constipation. These include: obstructions in the bowel, sometimes as a result of cancer; neurological diseases such as Parkinson's or multiple sclerosis, which interfere with nerve function; weak or tense pelvic muscles; conditions that disrupt hormone balance, such as an underactive or overactive thyroid or diabetes; and chronic inflammation. Treating these will improve colon function.

My Recommendations

Keep in mind that most constipation is not a disease that requires medications, but rather a symptom that requires some lifestyle correction. We fall into bad habits, such as rarely exercising, eating poorly, and not getting adequate amounts of fluids. These are some simple ways to correct the situation:

Chewing your food: One of the lost arts of eating, which was more often discussed when I was a young boy, was chewing your food thoroughly. Americans tend to eat too fast, and as a consequence, a significant portion of food goes undigested and eventually forms hard stools. Food should be chewed until it has a consistency of a liquid mush. This can go a long way in preventing constipation.

Exercise: The more active you are, the less likely you will suffer from chronic constipation. Sit-ups, running, brisk walking, and any exercise that requires contraction of abdominal and surrounding muscles will help reduce constipation.

Hydration: Chronic dehydration is one of the most common problems associated with chronic constipation, so become diligent about keeping well hydrated. Eating a lot of vegetables and some fruits can supply a good deal of water, as well as fiber. In addition, drink healthy beverages, such as white or green tea, purified water, and unsweetened drinks.

Drinking lots of vegetables: Turning green vegetables into a drink, by blending them with water or ice in a high-powered blender, is the best way to maximize your absorption of nutrients and fiber. Chapter 3 explains how to make such drinks. Have one or more glasses each day. After starting to do this, most people notice that their bowel movements significantly improve in consistency and frequency. The way you know your intake of green vegetables is adequate is that your stools will become green.

The combination of a high vegetable diet, good hydration, regular exercise, and taking daily magnesium supplements will almost guarantee you will not suffer from chronic constipation.

Natural Supplements

In general, I do not recommend using so-called "natural supplements" that stimulate colon contraction, as they can share some of the same side effects as pharmaceutical laxatives. These include aloe, senna, castor oil, and cascara sagrada.

The best natural laxatives contain both insoluble and soluble forms of fiber. The insoluble fibers add bulk, making it easier for the colon to pass the stool. In addition, insoluble fibers are fermented in the bowel and produce a number of compounds that promote intestinal health. For treating occasional constipation, consider one of these: psyllium, European buckthorn, inulin, guar gum, flaxseed fiber, or slippery elm.

Most important, I have found that one of the most overlooked causes of constipation, one that should always be addressed, is impaired digestion of foods. This is a common problem seen in the elderly, but is increasingly becoming more common in younger populations.

Although it may sound surprising, low stomach acid is often a problem, as is lack of digestive enzymes, which break down food. The lack of these result in food being poorly digested and hard stools being formed in the colon. Major digestive enzymes include lipases to digest fats, amylases for carbohydrates, and proteases for proteins. Supplements to replenish these, along with magnesium, will improve daily bowel movements.

▶ Digestive Enzymes and Acid Boosters

An enzyme supplement should contain a wide assortment of digestive enzymes, such as Digestive Enzymes Ultra, made by Pure Encapsulations. There are several ways to increase stomach acid, including drinking apple cider vinegar or pickle juice, or taking apple cider vinegar tablets or betaine HCL capsules.

➡ **What to do:** With each meal, take two capsules of Digestive Enzymes Ultra and apple cider vinegar (either one tablet or one teaspoon of pure, organic apple cider vinegar in a 4 ounce glass of water.) As an alternative to apple cider vinegar, you can take betaine HCL. The dose varies, depending on the severity of acid loss in the stomach. Start with one capsule of betaine HCL with a meal. At each meal after that, increase the dosage by one pill, until you feel warmth in your stomach. Once you feel this warmth, back off by one capsule until you no longer feel the warmth. If you have gastritis or an ulcer, do not take betaine HCL.

▶ Magnesium

Most people are magnesium deficient, especially those who eat a diet low in fruits and vegetables, the main natural sources of magnesium. Consequently, I recommend taking a magnesium supplement. Everyone notices that once they start taking magnesium, their bowel movements drastically improve, especially if they are elderly.

One of the problems with magnesium supplements is absorption. Most people will have difficulty absorbing magnesium oxide or magnesium sulfate, and as a consequence, they will develop diarrhea. Better absorbed forms, such as magnesium lactate, magnesium citrate, or magnesium malate are far less likely to produce diarrhea unless taken in excess, yet they will improve daily bowel movements. Time-release forms are most effective.

➡ **What to do:** I recommend taking Magnesium w/SRT, made by Jigsaw Health. It is a sustained, slow-release magnesium malate containing 500 mg of magnesium per four tablets, along with small amounts of vitamin C, folate, and methylcobalamin, the best form of vitamin B12. Take two tablets at bedtime (it also helps you sleep) and three tablets before breakfast. This will assure you will be regular.

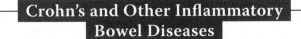

Crohn's and Other Inflammatory Bowel Diseases

Crohn's and ulcerative colitis are the two most common types of inflammatory bowel disease, and they share many symptoms. In Crohn's disease, the inflammation extends through the entire thickness of the intestine, whereas in ulcerative colitis, the inflammation is mainly centered in the mucosa, that is, along the surface of the inner colon. The severity and frequency of the attacks can vary widely.

In both cases, there is chronic or recurring inflammation in the digestive tract, as a result of a misguided immune response. The body's immune system is attacking its own gastrointestinal system, as though it were a pathogen. Both conditions share many common features and are associated with inflammation and damage to widespread areas of the body, including the central nervous system and nerves.

A less serious and less recognized form of inflammatory bowel disease is a condition called

---

SYMPTOMS OF CROHN'S AND ULCERATIVE COLITIS

The Crohn's and Colitis Foundation of America identified these as symptoms of inflammation in the digestive tract, which may appear with Crohn's or ulcerative colitis:

- Diarrhea
- Rectal bleeding
- Urgent need to move bowels
- Abdominal cramps and pain
- Sensation of incomplete evacuation
- Fever
- Constipation (can lead to bowel obstruction)
- Loss of appetite
- Weight loss
- Fatigue
- Night sweats
- Loss of normal menstrual cycle

Risk Factors

- Regular use of NSAIDs, such as ibuprofen or naproxen
- History of smoking, especially high in present smokers
- Use of birth control pills by women who smoke
- Previous viral intestinal infections or food poisoning
- An imbalance of gut bacteria

microscopic ulcerative colitis. It mostly affects middle-aged and elderly women who have smoked or are current smokers. The inflammation is less severe than in full-blown ulcerative colitis.

⌘ Conventional Treatment

Diagnosis of these conditions may include blood and stool tests, imaging tests, and/or a colonoscopy. Sometimes, long periods of remission occur for no known reason, but there is no known conventional cure. Medications may be used to reduce symptoms and, in severe cases, surgery may be done to remove part of the colon.

👍 My Recommendations

A considerable amount of data suggests that diet is playing a major role in these disorders. The highest incidence of inflammatory bowel diseases (IBD) is in the Western-developed nations. As the Western diet begins to invade the developing nations, we see a corresponding rise in IBD cases. Interestingly, the earliest disease to appear is ulcerative colitis and later Crohn's disease, suggesting that the longer one eats an unhealthy, Western diet, the worse the effect on the intestine. The Western diet is high in pro-inflammatory oils (omega-6 oils), high in protein, and extremely high in sugar, especially high fructose corn syrup—all things that are known to worsen inflammatory diseases.

A study done in Israel, in which the diet of 87 confirmed cases of IBD were analyzed, found that the strongest link was with a high intake of sugar, fat, and omega-6 oils, such as corn, safflower, sunflower, peanut, and soybean oils. Most processed foods, salad dressing, and baked products contain these oils.

Studies have shown that 98 percent of Crohn's patients have invasive E. coli bacteria in their colon. These nasty bacteria are also seen in 42 percent of patients with ulcerative colitis. Probiotics and colostrum help control such infection by inhibiting the growth of these invasive bacterial species.

Diet is essential in controlling both conditions. Chronic inflammation, especially involving the intestines, can cause a significant loss of nutrients, especially water-soluble B vitamins, vitamin C, magnesium, and zinc. Severe iron loss, especially seen with ulcerative colitis, can lead to severe anemia.

A modified Mediterranean diet, one without milk, other dairy products, or gluten, would be best. Most important is avoiding the omega-6 oils, such as corn, safflower, sunflower, peanut, soybean, and canola oils, as these increase inflammation. This means avoiding all foods fried in these oils and all salad dressings and processed foods made with any of them.

Instead of eating red meat, protein should come from eggs, chicken, turkey, and possibly pork. It is best if meats are eaten only two to three times a week. The ideal diet should consist mostly of vegetables, especially those that are high in nutrients, such as broccoli, Brussels sprouts, cauliflower, cabbage, kale, and other leafy greens. Making these into a drink, as described in chapter 3, would be best.

Before deciding on a diet, it's best to be tested for food allergies and intolerances, which can be a lot more subtle than outright food allergies. For detecting food intolerances, the Alcat test appears to be one of the best.

Natural Supplements

Supplements can help to rebalance the immune system, calm inflammation, and soothe symptoms. Taken regularly, they can also help to heal damage in the gastrointestinal tract.

▶ Curcumin

Curcumin is a powerful anti-inflammatory, antioxidant, and antimicrobial substance extracted from turmeric, the curry spice. Lab, animal, and human research shows that it cools dendritic cells, which are one of the central activators of inflammation in inflammatory bowel diseases. Curcumin also reduces inflammatory chemicals released by immune cells, which are major players in inflammatory intestinal diseases.

In one such study, researchers used 89 patients with ulcerative colitis. They were divided into 45 patients given curcumin and 44 patients given a placebo. One of the worst effects of ulcerative colitis is recurrent bouts of severe abdominal pain and bloody diarrhea. They found that the patients receiving curcumin had threefold fewer recurrences than those getting the placebo. After one year, the episodes were much less intense among curcumin users, and colonoscopies showed that their colons looked much healthier than those taking a placebo.

➡ **What to do:** Curcumin is poorly absorbed as a powder in a capsule, but when mixed with an oil, such as extra virgin olive oil or coconut oil, absorption improves up to 11-fold. Break open capsules of powdered curcumin, mix with a teaspoon of the oil, and swallow. I find that it dissolves much better in warm coconut oil. Take 250 mg to 500 mg, three times a day, with meals. As an alternative, take capsules that are specially formulated to be absorbable: CurcumaSorb, made by Pure Encapsulations. One capsule contains 250 mg.

▶ Hesperidin

Hesperidin is in the same family of nutrients as curcumin, called flavonoids, but is very well absorbed and distributed throughout the body, including the brain. Animal studies have shown that hesperidin can significantly reduce the colon inflammation in ulcerative colitis. Because it is so well absorbed, it would also be very useful in treating Crohn's disease.

➡ **What to do:** Take 500 to 1,000 mg, three times a day, with meals.

▶ Naringenin

Naringenin is a flavonoid compound found in high concentrations in grapefruit. It has powerful anti-inflammatory properties.

In addition, one of its main benefits is preventing damage to the intestinal barrier, which is always damaged early on during inflammatory bowel diseases.

Intestinal cells are arranged very close together, in what is called a tight junction, and this arrangement prevents large food particles and microorganisms from entering the blood stream from the gut. When the gut barrier is damaged, we call it a leaky gut, because food particles pass into the blood stream and increase inflammation and autoimmune reactions. Animal studies show that naringenin plays a major role in preventing this from happening and in repairing leaky gut.

➡ **What to do:** Take 500 mg, three times a day, with meals.

▶ Berberine

This compound has been used for hundreds of years to treat gastrointestinal disorders. Studies have shown that, like naringenin, berberine can prevent disruption of the intestinal barrier and reduce inflammation in the intestines.

➡ **What to do:** Take 400 mg, two to three times a day, with meals.

▶ Colostrum

This is the watery fluid that is secreted by the breast just before milk is released. It plays a major role in immune function and gut health in the newborn baby. Recent studies have found that it can also help adults with inflammatory gut problems. It heals the leaky gut that is associated with all inflammatory bowel diseases. I recommend using a high-quality colostrum supplement, such as Colostrum LD capsules, made by Sovereign Laboratories.

➡ **What to do:** Take one to two capsules, three times a day, with meals. The product instructions recommend taking it between meals, but I find less stomach upset if you take it with meals, and studies show that it is effective when taken with food.

▶ Omega-3 Fish Oil

These oils contain two major components, EPA and DHA, both of which reduce inflammation by separate mechanisms. Some products contain both of these and others contain only one.

➡ **What to do:** Take either 1,000 mg of DHA twice a day with meals or 2,000 to 3,000 mg daily of an EPA-DHA combination, such as Carlson's fish oil—a flavored liquid version, orange or lemon, makes it easy to take a large dose and tastes quite good. If you have intense symptoms, take the combination form.

▶ Magnesium

Magnesium is essential for the operation of several hundred enzymes in cells, is an anti-inflammatory, and improves blood flow through blood vessels. Equally important, it reduces excitotoxicity (described in chapter 2), which occurs in the intestines with exposure to dietary glutamate or aspartame.

I have found magnesium to be very effective in treating intestinal cramping, especially associated with food poisoning and other inflammatory bowel diseases. There are different forms of magnesium, and poorly absorbed ones, such as magnesium oxide and magnesium sulfate, can cause severe diarrhea. Magnesium citrate, malate, or a combination of the two is better absorbed. I prefer a slow-release form, such as Magnesium w/SRT, made by Jigsaw Health.

➡ **What to do:** Take two slow-release magnesium malate tablets twice daily, with meals. This will supply a total of 500 mg of magnesium. Chronic inflammation anywhere in the body can cause extensive loss of magnesium, and the exact best dose depends on one's blood levels and the severity of the disease.

▶ Zinc

Zinc is another mineral frequently lost with inflammatory bowel diseases, especially Crohn's disease. Zinc reduces inflammation and is vital for tissue strength and metabolism.

➡ **What to do:** Take 30 mg of zinc picolinate, once daily.

▶ Vitamin D3

Vitamin D3 is produced in the inner layers of the skin, upon exposure to direct rays of the sun. Very little vitamin D is supplied by the diet. It is an immune modulator, meaning that when the immune system is overacting it calms the reaction and, if deficient, it improves immunity. It also plays a major role in protecting the brain. Oral replacement requires rather high doses. The dose seen in most supplements—400 IU a day—has been shown to have no effect on blood levels of the vitamin.

> ➡ **What to do:** Before taking vitamin D3 as a supplement, your blood vitamin D3 level should be tested. This is a common test. The optimum level is between 65 ng/ml and 95 ng/ml. The dose needed depends on the degree of deficiency.
>
> If the level is less than 30 ng/ml, the dose is 10,000 IU of vitamin D3 a day, taken with a meal, for three weeks, and then repeat the blood test. Once blood levels are in the target range, reduce the daily dose to 5,000 IU.
>
> If the blood level is between 35 and 50 ng/ml, I recommend taking 5,000 IU a day for three weeks and then repeating the blood test. If levels are within the optimum range, reduce the dose to 2,000 IU a day. Babies can take 1,000 IU a day and toddlers and small children can take 2,000 IU a day.

▶ B Vitamins

The B-vitamins, such as thiamine, riboflavin, pantothenic acid, niacinamide, and biotin, are quickly lost from the body with chronic inflammation and stress, both present with IBD disorders.

> ➡ **What to do:** Take a balanced multivitamin/mineral supplement daily, such as Extend Core, made by Vitamin Research Products. It is a well-balanced formula, although it

does not contain iron. Take two capsules of Extend Core, three times a day, with meals.

▶ Iron

Iron is depleted during chronic inflammation, and in the case of inflammatory bowel diseases, iron loss can be significant, especially with ulcerative colitis, which has bloody diarrhea. Over time, severe iron-deficiency anemia can result. It is important to have a complete iron panel test done that includes free iron, transferrin, ferritin, and iron binding capacity.

The best iron supplement is carbonyl iron. Unlike most other iron supplements, it softens stools, rather than causing constipation, and is well absorbed without causing stomach upset.

➡ **What to do:** The dose depends on the severity of the iron loss. For mild to moderate iron-deficiency anemia, the daily dose for adults is 3 mg per kilogram body weight, with a meal. For severe iron-deficiency anemia, the daily dose is 6 mg per kilogram of body weight. Some people have a lot of difficulty absorbing iron. In that case, take 250 to 500 mg of vitamin C along with the iron supplement.

▶ Hyperbaric Oxygen Therapy (HBOT)

Some studies have been done using HBOT to treat inflammatory bowel diseases, such as Crohn's disease and ulcerative colitis. These have shown improvement in symptoms and tests that measure bowel inflammation.

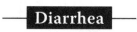

Diarrhea

Also simply called "the runs," diarrhea is medically defined as having loose, watery stools more than three times in one day. Other symptoms may include an urgent need to go to the bathroom, bloating, nausea, or cramps. In children, the condition can be dangerous, and if it lasts more than two days, a doctor should be consulted.

Even among adults, diarrhea merits medical attention if it lasts more than five days or is severe and lasts more than three days; brings about weakness or dehydration; or is accompanied by severe pain, fever, or blood in the stools. Chronic or recurring diarrhea can be a symptom of other conditions. See the sections, "Inflammatory Bowel Diseases" and "Irritable Bowel Syndrome" for more details.

A number of prescription drugs can cause diarrhea, including acid-lowering medications such as Tagamet, Zantac, and Axid; ibuprofen; and proton-pump inhibitors such as Nexium and Prilosec. In some cases, the diarrhea is severe.

Travelers' diarrhea can be caused by contamination of food or water with various bacteria or parasites. And, intestinal parasites can occur and cause chronic diarrhea in anyone, without travel. In such situations, comprehensive stool testing is required to make a diagnosis.

> **DIARRHEA TRIGGERS**
>
> Although causes of diarrhea are not always known, these are some possible ones:
> - Food poisoning
> - Viral infection
> - Lactose intolerance
> - Soy intolerance
> - Some antibiotics
> - Chemotherapy drugs
> - Gluten intolerance
> - Celiac disease
> - Candida colon overgrowth
> - Irritable bowel syndrome
> - Crohn's disease
> - AIDS or HIV
> - Malabsorption of fats

Conventional Treatment

Drinking plenty of fluids to avoid dehydration is a basic step in home care, as well as trying to identify any foods that may have triggered diarrhea, and avoiding them. Medically, hydration is a key step, and may be done with intravenous fluids if the condition is severe. Over-the-counter diarrhea medication may also be recommended.

Other treatment depends upon whether there is an identifiable cause of the diarrhea. For example, it could be a side effect of a medication, or a symptom of an underlying condition. If it is related to a chronic condition, such as irritable bowel syndrome (see the separate section on this), lifestyle changes may be recommended.

👍 My Recommendations

Generally, these are the most effective steps to take for acute diarrhea:

- Avoid solid foods until your bowel movements return to normal.

- Keep well hydrated—drink at least three 12-ounce glasses of purified water or decaffeinated tea three times a day. Decaffeinated white or green tea can reduce the level of dangerous, diarrhea-causing bacteria and calm inflammation within the intestinal lining.

- Avoid caffeine.

- Avoid dairy products. Diarrhea can induce temporary lactose deficiency and this can worsen the diarrhea.

Chronic or recurring diarrhea is a serious symptom that should not be ignored but should be discussed with your physician. For example, it can be a symptom of a serious condition in the intestines, such as Crohn's disease or ulcerative colitis, a systemic disease such as hyperthyroidism, or gluten intolerance or Celiac disease, which requires a gluten-free diet.

🐇 Natural Supplements

For the occasional bout of diarrhea, relief can come with a number of supplements and foods, such as colostrum, zinc, slippery elm, chamomile tea, blueberries, or carob. For small children and infants, add one to two teaspoons of carob to their food, two to three times a day.

When there is no serious disease, the most common cause of diarrhea is dysbiosis—abnormal growth of bacteria in the colon. Often, it develops following a course of antibiotics, which kill beneficial bacteria in the colon, as well as harmful ones. These beneficial bacteria have a number of functions, including reducing inflammation in the body and suppressing the growth of harmful bacteria and yeast. In addition, most people eat meat of animals fed antibiotics, and antibiotics may be in their tap water.

▶ Probiotics

Another name for beneficial bacteria, probiotics are available in many supplements. They can replenish the natural beneficial bacteria in the digestive system and control future growth of harmful bacteria. It's important to choose a high-quality product that contains a variety of live organisms in adequate amounts.

Studies have shown that different types of bacteria provide different health benefits. For example, Lactobacillus casei species has been shown to greatly improve the production of secretory IgA, a protective antibody released along the inside of the intestine. People with low intestinal IgA experience numerous infections and food intolerances. In my practice, when I did comprehensive stool testing on patients, I rarely saw a person with adequate numbers of these essential organisms.

An adequate probiotic should contain the following bacteria with a population of at least 5 billion each:

Bifidobacterium species

- B. lactis
- B. bifidum
- B. infantis
- B. longus

Lactobacillus species

- L. acidophilus

- L. brevis

- L. bulgaricus

- L. paracasei

- L. rhamnosus

- L. casei

I recommend buying a refrigerated product with a guarantee of its potency.

➡ **What to do:** Take two capsules of a product containing no less than 5 billion organisms, once a week. If you are taking antibiotics, before your start, take two capsules of a supplement that contains at least 50 billion live organisms. Take this dose throughout your treatment and continue with one capsule daily for the next three weeks. Then go back to your maintenance dose of two capsules a week. An excellent brand is the Garden of Life formulation by Dr. David Perlmutter, which contains 90 billion organisms.

Food Poisoning

Food poisoning affects millions of Americans each year, and though it most often resolves on its own, it can become serious, or even deadly, in some instances. The poison can be any type of pathogen that found its way into food through spoilage or errors in food processing facilities, including toxins such as chemicals, bacteria, viruses, parasites, or other infectious particles.

Conventional Treatment

Getting plenty of fluids, along with rest, is the most important treatment, and often is enough for the condition to pass. However, any of these symptoms indicate a need for medical help: fever, lightheadedness or weakness as a result of dehydration, diarrhea that lasts more than 72 hours, or vomiting that prevents fluids from being replaced. Medical treatment may include hydration and medications to control vomiting and diarrhea. Although uncommon, vascular collapse, which means a loss of blood pressure and eventual cardiac failure, is one of the most dangerous side effects of food poisoning. Coagulation of the blood in arteries of the extremities can also occur, and can lead to amputations. Fortunately, such complications are quite rare.

👍 My Recommendations

On one occasion, I was stricken with severe food poisoning and was so sick, I had to lie on the floor, sweating profusely, gripped by waves of intense pain. I remembered that magnesium was an excellent relaxant for smooth muscles, and so I made my usual magnesium solution by adding 250 mg of magnesium citrate powder to 12 ounces of water. By the time I had finished drinking the mixture, my pain began to subside considerably and within three minutes, I was pain-free. I have since recommended this treatment to others, who have had similar success.

COMMON SYMPTOMS OF FOOD POISONING
• Stomach cramping
• Nausea
• Vomiting
• Diarrhea
These commonly lead to dehydration, which can become dangerous.

Once the attack is over, the lining of the stomach and intestine is still inflamed and this needs to be addressed. Avoid soups, especially those containing MSG or other food additives with glutamate, as this stimulates the glutamate receptors lining the intestines and can trigger intense spasms and diarrhea. It is important to drink plenty of filtered water—at least 24 ounces over the next hour. You can add magnesium citrate to the water (250 mg to each 12 ounces). This will further calm the pain.

One of the major sources of food contamination is food handlers having infected cuts on their hands. All food handlers should wear gloves. For meals prepared at home, never use wooden cutting boards, and surfaces should be cleaned after meat has been on them. Hands should be thoroughly washed after handling any raw meat product.

In my opinion, all meats should be cooked thoroughly, as most meats are contaminated with some bacteria and viruses. Tasting meats, such as ground beef, before they are fully cooked is a recipe for disaster.

Natural Supplements

▶ Magnesium

The right type of magnesium can bring relief from even severe reactions to food poisoning. Daily magnesium supplements can shore up the internal defenses to toxins and pathogens in food, and if food poisoning does occur, the symptoms will be less extreme.

➡ **What to do:** For acute attacks of food poisoning, immediately drink a mixture of 1 scoop (250 mg) of Magnesium Powder (a citrate form), made by Pure Encapsulations, in 12 ounces of filtered water. This can be repeated as necessary, but usually a single treatment suffices. To reduce the risk of severe reactions to food poisoning, take a daily supplement of a slow-release form of magnesium malate called Magnesium w/SRT, made by Jigsaw Health. Take two caplets, two to three times a day.

▶ Apigenin

This is a natural flavonoid found in celery and parsley. A number of studies have shown that it quiets intestinal inflammation.

➡ **What to do:** Take two capsules (100 mg), three times a day of Apigenin, made by Swanson. For severe cases, the dose can be increased to four capsules (200 mg), three times a day.

▶ Luteolin

A flavonoid found in celery and artichokes luteolin is a powerful antioxidant and reduces inflammation in inflammatory bowel disorders. Luteolin Complex, made by Swanson, is a good product.

➧ **What to do:** Take one capsule (100 mg), three times a day with meals. For severe cases, increase the dose to three capsules, three times a day with meals.

Gallstones

Gallstones form in the gallbladder, a small organ in the upper right of the abdominal area, just below the rib cage. The gallbladder is a little sac that stores bile, a fluid made by the liver to aid in the breakdown and digestion of fats, cholesterol, and fat-soluble vitamins. After fat is eaten, the gallbladder contracts and secretes bile, through a duct, into the small intestine, where it is used in digestion. Although gallstones often cause no discomfort, they may cause bloating, cramps, fever, nausea, and pain, sometimes to an excruciating degree. Gallbladder disease can be acute or chronic, with recurring bouts of pain. Symptoms that appear within 30 minutes to an hour after eating fatty or fried food are a telltale sign.

> **WHO IS AT RISK?**
>
> It's estimated that 20 percent of Americans may have gallstones but only 1 to 3 percent experience symptoms of pain or other discomfort. Gallstones most often develop in overweight, middle-aged women but the most severe symptoms occur among men and the elderly. These can increase risk:
>
> - Being overweight or obese
> - Crash diets that lead to sudden weight loss
> - Birth control pills
> - Cholesterol-lowering medications

Most gallstones are composed of cholesterol and can vary in size from a single large stone to many smaller ones. There may be no symptoms. Trouble occurs when these stones travel out of the gallbladder and get stuck in the bile duct leading to the small intestine. In such cases, severe pain is common and stools may have a white or pale appearance. Blockage of the bile duct can turn urine dark and lead to serious complications, including jaundice, rupture of the gallbladder, which can be deadly, and an inflamed pancreas (see the "Pancreatitis" section).

Pain caused by impacted gallstones typically occurs in the right upper quadrant of the abdomen, just below the ribs. It can also extend to the back, just under the shoulder blade, or to the breastbone in the center of the chest. Recurrent nausea and gas after meals can indicate gallbladder problems. There is evidence that when gallstones form, there is inflammation within the gallbladder.

Conventional Treatment

Diagnosis of gallstones usually includes a blood test to rule out kidney disease, an ultrasound, and sometimes a special type of x-ray or CT scan. Treatment depends upon the individual situation. Gallstones that produce no symptoms generally require no treatment. When they are problematic, there is no permanent medical cure, and in extreme cases, the gallbladder may be removed. However, gallbladder removal is fraught with complications and long-term digestive problems. Most gallbladder disease can be treated with dietary changes and rest.

My Recommendations

Avoiding obesity will reduce the risk of gallbladder disease and gallstones. High-fat diets, especially those containing omega-6 oils, such as corn, soy, and cottonseed oils, often lead to gallbladder problems because they trigger inflammation. By following a diet high in vegetables, low in sugars, and moderate in meats, gallbladder problems are much less likely. Preventing and reducing chronic inflammation is the most important objective, as inflammation appears to play the major role.

A high-vegetable diet is anti-inflammatory. In addition, animal studies have shown that garlic and onions both inhibit and dissolve gallstones, and raw and dried extracts of these are effective.

🐇 Natural Supplements

▶ Magnesium

Magnesium is a major inhibitor of inflammation and spasms associated with gallstones impacted in the bile ducts. Acute attacks of gallstone pain can be quickly stopped by drinking magnesium mixed in water. Daily magnesium supplements can help to prevent attacks.

➡ **What to do:** For acute gallstone pain, immediately drink a mixture of one scoop (250 mg) of Magnesium Powder (a citrate form), made by Pure Encapsulations, in 12 ounces of filtered water. To reduce the risk of gallstone attacks, take a daily supplement of a slow-release form of magnesium malate called Magnesium w/SRT, made by Jigsaw Health. Take two caplets, two to three times a day.

▶ Curcumin

Curcumin is a powerful anti-inflammatory compound found in higher concentrations in the curry spice turmeric. Curcumin increases bile flow, thus reducing the risk of forming stones. However, if stones are impacted in the bile duct, it might worsen the pain. Studies using massive doses found it to have a very high margin of overall safety.

➡ **What to do:** Take 250 to 500 mg, three times a day, with meals. Use a highly absorbable form such as CurcumaSorb, made by Pure Encapsulations. Or, to improve absorption of powdered curcumin supplements, mix the powder contents of a capsule with a tablespoon of coconut or extra virgin olive oil. This can be messy.

▶ Luteolin

A flavonoid found in celery and artichokes luteolin is a powerful antioxidant and reduces inflammation in digestive disorders. It has been shown to inhibit gallstone formation and protect the health of the bile ducts. Luteolin Complex, made by Swanson, is a good product.

➡ **What to do:** Take one capsule (100 mg), three times a day with meals. For severe cases, increase the dose to three capsules, three times a day with meals.

▶ EPA

The EPA component of fish oil significantly inhibits the formation of gallstones. The other major fish oil component, DHA, has only mild effects. Fish oil naturally contains both components, but some products are made with high amounts of one or the other. If your objective is to prevent or treat gallstones, Elite EPA Gems, made by Carlson, is a good high-EPA product. It contains 1,000 mg of EPA in one capsule.

➡ **What to do:** Take one capsule daily of Elite EPA Gems.

▶ Garlic Extract

There are a number of higher quality garlic extracts. One is Kyolic Aged Garlic Extract, made by Wakunaga, and another is GarliActive, made by Pure Encapsulations.

➡ **What to do:** Take 600 mg, twice a day, of either garlic extract.

— Gas —

We usually think of gas as flatulence but it can also manifest as belching or burping. It's normal for some gas to develop during the digestive process, as bacteria in the gut break down food, and most of the time, it has no odor. The release of gas is a normal part of healthy digestion. Swallowing air along with food also contributes to gas.

While it can be annoying in excess, gas usually doesn't require medical attention, unless accompanied by other symptoms, such as stomach or rectal pain, nausea or vomiting, constipation, heartburn, diarrhea, fever, unexplained weight loss, or stools that are bloody or have a strong odor.

GAS FACTS

Most people pass gas between 13 and 21 times each day, as flatulence or through the mouth as belches or burps. Common triggers of excess gas include:

- Eating too quickly
- Drinking fizzy beverages
- Chewing gum
- Dairy products
- Beans
- Cabbage
- Antibiotics
- Digestive problems

Conventional Treatment

Where gas becomes a significant problem and doesn't resolve by itself, or is combined with other symptoms, a doctor is likely to check what foods you are eating, to see if there are one or more triggers, and may look for any underlying conditions. Tests may include special x-rays or scans, blood tests, and an abdominal ultrasound. Treatment may be as simple as some dietary changes or may be more comprehensive, depending upon the diagnosis.

My Recommendations

A number of foods are naturally associated with producing intestinal gas, such as broccoli, Brussels sprouts, cauliflower, cabbage, and beans. Soaking beans overnight with an added onion can reduce the chemical that causes the gas. This can be time-consuming, but works. After cooking the beans, pour off the water.

Natural Supplements

Incomplete digestion of food, especially starches, can cause gas. This is where the digestive enzymes come in handy. See the Constipation section for how to use enzyme supplements.

▶ Activated Charcoal

If you know that you will be eating gas-producing foods, plan on taking activated charcoal tablets to prevent problems. Charcoal won't work if you take it a few hours after a meal.

➡ **What to do:** Take one or two capsules at the start of the meal, but don't do this daily as it will rob you of minerals. Never take activated charcoal with medication, as it can absorb the medication.

▶ Magnesium

Attacks of gas pains can be relieved by taking magnesium citrate or magnesium citrate and/or malate in water. The magnesium reduces inflammation and calms intestinal muscle spasms. I have also found it to be very useful for treating intestinal cramping associated with food poisoning.

➡ **What to do:** Mix two capsules of the magnesium (250 mg per capsule) in a 12-ounce glass of water and drink. Or, mix a powdered magnesium supplement in water.

▶ Peppermint and Ginger Teas

In between meals, a strong cup of peppermint tea can reduce gas pains, but do not take it within an hour of eating. Peppermint relaxes the valve in the lower esophagus that keeps food in the stomach and when combined with food, can trigger acid reflux. Ginger tea, which you can drink with your meal, can also help to relieve gas.

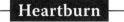

Heartburn

Heartburn and acid reflux are two sides of the same coin. Heartburn is the burning or irritation we sometimes feel after eating. Acid reflux, and GERD (Gastroesophageal reflux disease), describe a malfunction in the digestive process that causes the sensation of heartburn.

After food goes down the esophagus, the tube that connects the mouth and the stomach, it is supposed to remain in the stomach, where digestive juices, including stomach acid, break it down. A ring-shaped muscle, the lower esophageal sphincter, is designed to close and seal the top of the stomach, but sometimes, it allows some partially digested food to move back up the esophagus, causing irritation and burning.

One of the most common causes of acid reflux is overeating and poor digestion of the food in the stomach. Americans tend to eat large meals, especially in some restaurants, and they eat their meals rapidly. Chewing is important for allowing the food to mix with the digestive juices and stomach acid, so as to allow the softened food to move on into the small intestine. Poorly chewed foods, especially meats, tend to stay in the stomach longer and can force the acid-mixed food into the lower esophagus, where it causes a burning sensation.

> **HEARTBURN TRIGGERS**
>
> These are some common conditions that increase the odds of heartburn:
>
> - Obesity
> - Smoking
> - Hiatal hernia
> - Pregnancy
> - Scleroderma (an autoimmune disease)
> - Drinking alcohol
> - Large amounts of abdominal fat (abdominal obesity)

Chronic acid reflux increases the risk of esophageal cancer. Studies have shown that the acid can also reflux as far as the vocal cords, leading to cancer there as well.

Conventional Treatment

Antacids and heartburn medications reduce the level of stomach acid. The drugs considered to be most effective are proton pump inhibitors, such as Prevacid, Prilosec, and Nexium. They inhibit a molecule known as a "gastric acid pump" that produces acid in the stomach, but side effects may include elevated blood pressure, damage to the heart, magnesium deficiency, and higher risk of hip fractures, notably when the drugs are used for more than two or three months.

Other drugs, known as H2 antagonists, block stomach acid through a different mechanism and don't have the same side effects but are considered less effective. These include Zantac, Tagamet, and Pepcid. These drugs are also associated with some dangerous complications. In some cases, surgery is recommended to correct the function of the lower esophageal sphincter muscle.

👍 My Recommendations

It's critically important to chew your food well, which means chewing until the food is a soft mush. Also avoid large meals and eating close to bedtime. It is important to avoid lying down after a meal, as this increases the likelihood that the acid-mixed food will reflux into the esophagus. After eating, wait at least two hours before lying down. Reflux is also more likely if you lay on your right side.

Drinking plenty of liquids with meals will dilute what little acid enters the esophagus, reducing the burning sensation. Avoid eating any mint containing peppermint, as it causes relaxation of the lower esophageal sphincter and increases the likelihood that stomach acid will reflux into the esophagus.

🐇 Natural Supplements

The most successful treatment I have seen is to increase stomach acid after a meal. This may seem counterintuitive, but studies have shown that low stomach acid is more common with acid reflux disease, rather than high levels of acid. What appears to be happening is that because the stomach's acid level is low, the enzymes needed to digest food, especially for proteins, cannot be activated, and this prevents the food from being digested. As a result, the food stays in the stomach. And with large meals in particular, the stomach becomes overfilled and food spills up into the lower esophagus. Even though the acid level is low, it is high enough to burn the delicate tissues of the esophagus.

So, you may be thinking, why do antacid medications seem to make me feel better—at least for a while? These medications lower the acid level so low that less burning occurs. Yet, over time, things actually get worse because most of your food is poorly digested and the upward pressure into the lower esophagus continues. The goal is to increase the level of stomach acid and improve food digestion. This is how it is done.

▶ Stomach Acid Boosters

To improve digestion, stomach acid can be enhanced with any of these:

- Take a tablespoon of pickle juice with each meal.

- Add a tablespoon of apple cider vinegar to 4 ounces of water and drink with each meal.

- Take two apple cider vinegar tablets with each meal.

▶ DGL

Short for deglycyrrhizinated licorice, DGL is a form of licorice that is excellent for soothing acute attacks of heartburn, by coating the lower esophagus and reducing the burning and damage caused by stomach acid. There are many chewable forms of DGL. I like a product called DGL Plus, made by Pure Encapsulations.

➡ **What to do:** To coat the esophagus, empty two capsules of DGL Plus in 4 ounces of water and drink between meals.

▶ Chewing Gum

Chewing gum can increase saliva production about eight or nine times higher than normal, helping to reduce the burning and damage caused by stomach acid. I would not use regular, sugared gum. A good alternative would be mastic gum, chewed after meals to reduce acid reflux damage.

▶ Protect Your Esophagus from Cancer

One of the most feared complications of chronic acid reflux is esophageal cancer. The above steps will reduce your risk, but a powerful added step is to take some supplements that reduce inflammation, have powerful anticancer effects, and promote healing of the esophagus.

▶ Curcumin and Quercetin

Both are anti-inflammatory and curcumin also increases production of saliva. Both are fat soluble, so both are absorbed most efficiently when the contents of capsules are mixed with fat. The combination will coat your esophagus and stomach. Do not use curcumin or quercetin products that are mixed with other compounds, as they will not dissolve properly.

➡ **What to do:** Break open capsules and mix one tablespoon of coconut oil or extra virgin olive oil with 250 mg curcumin powder and 250 mg quercetin powder. Take once daily.

▶ Apigenin

This is a flavonoid found in some vegetables. It has been shown to significantly reduce inflammation in the gastrointestinal tract.

➡ **What to do:** Take 100 mg, three times a day, with meals.

Irritable Bowel Syndrome

Irritable bowel syndrome, or IBS, affects one in six Americans at some time in life, and twice as many women as men. Its causes are not fully understood, but recent research suggests that, in some people, it may be a milder or early form of inflammatory bowel disease. The intestinal muscles are hyperactive in their reaction to many normal stimuli, resulting in symptoms such as bowel distention after a meal. There are far more people with the condition than are being diagnosed by physicians, but many cases are simply dismissed as other problems.

IBS is classified into these major subtypes:

- IBS-C: has frequent constipation

- IBS-D: diarrhea is more frequent

- IBS-M: a mixed form, with alternating bouts of constipation and diarrhea

- IBS-U: has no particular pattern of stool abnormalities

Many physicians diagnose IBS as a problem affecting depressed people, especially women. Depression, especially when combined with anxiety, is very common with IBS, but it appears that the medical profession has things backwards: IBS is not caused by depression, rather, the depression is caused by inflammation related to IBS. When the intestines are inflamed, the brain becomes instantly inflamed as well, and this manifests as depression and/or anxiety. The gut is linked to the brain by the vagus nerve, the longest nerve extending from the brain stem to the abdomen, and neurological symptoms from IBS can occur quite rapidly.

> **IBS SYMPTOMS**
>
> The main symptoms are:
> - Stomach pain
> - Gas
> - A sensation of fullness
> - Bloating
> - Diarrhea
> - Constipation
> - Alternating diarrhea and constipation

A leaky gut is common with both IBS and IBD (inflammatory bowel disease). This leakiness allows large particles of food to enter the bloodstream, where these can trigger immune reactions producing long-term inflammation. The inflammation magnifies pain signals, leading to intensely painful IBS spasms.

⭐ Conventional Treatment

There is no medical test for IBS, but blood and stool tests, x-rays, and/or a colonoscopy may be done to rule out other known diseases. If there is an underlying intestinal infection, it can be treated with antibiotics, but otherwise, medications can only reduce or mask symptoms, such as constipation, diarrhea, intestinal spasms, or pain.

Lifestyle changes are sometimes suggested but since triggers differ among individuals, there is no single prescribed regimen. Doctors may recommend avoiding stimulating substances, such as caffeine in coffee, tea, and sodas, and eating smaller meals.

👍 My Recommendations

Various things can lead to inflammation that triggers IBS. These include infections in the intestines, food poisoning, pro-inflammatory foods such as omega-6 oils (including corn, safflower, sunflower, peanut, and soybean oils), high sugar intake, and glutamate food additives.

Chapter 2 contains more information about glutamate. Briefly, as a food additive, it is an excitotoxin, meaning it overstimulates cells, causing cellular harm and death. A great many processed foods contain glutamate additives. MSG (monosodium glutamate) is the most obvious form but there are many others, listed in chapter 2. Research shows that glutamate food additives can overstimulate the nerves and muscles of the digestive tract, leading to intestinal cramping, excess stomach acid, and abnormal release of digestive enzymes, and they can worsen all the symptoms of IBS.

In addition, many foods naturally contain significant amounts of glutamate that can make IBS worse when eaten in excess, especially when the food is processed, fermented, or slow cooked. In general, raw whole foods, even though they may contain significant levels of glutamate, are safe because the glutamate is released slowly, thus preventing an overload of glutamate in the blood stream. Liquid forms of excitotoxins, such as glutamate in soy sauce and aspartic acid in aspartame-sweetened juices, are rapidly absorbed and more harmful. Here are some foods that are high in glutamate:

- All meats, but especially red meats

- Meat gravies and meat-based sauces

- All mushrooms, but especially portobello mushrooms

- All cheeses, but especially parmesan and gorgonzola cheeses

- Packaged sauces, especially white and tomato sauces

- Powdered and pureed tomatoes (whole tomatoes are generally safe)

- Many nuts, especially peanuts, cashews, and walnuts. These also contain many beneficial substances and minerals, and should be eaten only in moderation. Be warned that some brands of peanuts contain added MSG.

For more information go to http://www.truthinlabeling.org.

Natural Supplements

Studies have shown that compared to healthy people, those suffering from IBS have abnormal quantities and species of bacteria in their colon. Beneficial bacteria, or probiotics, play a vital role in reducing inflammation in the intestines, and in the entire body, so correcting probiotic deficiencies is one of the most important things that can be done for IBS. See the "Diarrhea" section for more details about using probiotics.

In addition, these supplements can help.

▶ Encapsulated Peppermint Oil

One of the best-studied natural treatments, reported in medical journals, is the use of enteric-coated peppermint capsules. These are designed to survive stomach acid and release peppermint oil in the intestine. The oil contains several unique nutrients, called flavonoids, that relax the intestinal tract, thus reducing the painful spasms and bloating associated with IBS.

In one such study, 40 patients taking peppermint capsules experienced these dramatic improvements:

- 79 percent had less abdominal pain

- 29 percent were pain-free

- 83 percent had less abdominal distention

- 83 percent had less frequent stools

- 73 percent had less intestinal rumbling

- 79 percent had less flatulence

These results were significantly better than for those receiving a placebo. Other studies have confirmed that peppermint capsules significantly reduce the pain of IBS and improve quality of life.

➡ **What to do:** Make sure capsules are enteric-coated and designed to release peppermint oil in the intestine. Take one capsule, three times daily, either one hour before eating or two hours after eating. Do not take capsules with meals or chew them, as they will release the peppermint into the esophagus and this will worsen reflux. Those with severe reflux may not be able to tolerate peppermint capsules, but they are worth a try. One commonly used brand is Heather's Tummy Tamers, which also contains fennel and ginger.

▶ Apigenin and Luteolin

These are both naturally present flavonoids and have been shown to reduce inflammatory bowel disease. Luteolin is found in peppermint and may explain some of its benefits. When tested in animals, apigenin has been shown to powerfully prevent autoimmune reactions, such as lupus. Apigenin is found in high concentrations in peppermint, parsley, thyme, olives, and chamomile. It may be one reason why peppermint works so well. It is not absorbed well from food sources, but the concentrated forms in supplement capsules are effective.

▶ **What to do:** Take 100 mg of apigenin and 100 to 200 mg of luteolin, three times daily with meals. Taking them together improves results.

▶ Hesperidin

This extract is in the flavonoid category of nutrients and is found in high concentrations in oranges. Hesperidin is a natural relaxant and antianxiety agent and reduces intestinal inflammation. One study found that people with IBS have more efficient absorption of hesperidin.

▶ **What to do:** Take 250 mg, three times daily with meals.

▶ Hyperbaric Oxygen Therapy (HBOT)

I am not aware of any studies on the use of HBOT for irritable bowel syndrome. However, because inflammation plays a significant role in this disorder and HBOT reduces inflammation, one would expect improvement.

Pancreatitis

An inflammation of the pancreas, pancreatitis may be acute or chronic. The two main causes are alcohol abuse and gallstones, and others include heredity, medications, injury, high triglyceride levels, and infection. However, it's estimated that the cause is unknown in as many as one-third of cases.

A large gland behind the stomach, the pancreas secretes enzymes into the small intestine to break down food, and produces two hormones—insulin and glucagon. These hormones enable carbohydrates to be converted into energy and regulate levels of blood sugar. When untreated and severe, pancreatitis can harm the liver, kidneys, lungs, heart, and other organs. Chronic pancreatitis increases one's risk of pancreatic cancer.

Conventional Treatment

Medical treatment aims to reduce inflammation and allow the pancreas to heal, and most cases of acute pancreatitis can be cured. Alcohol should always be avoided. Sometimes, a liquid diet is used for one or two days. Generally, a low-fat diet with plenty of fluids is recommended, and enzymes may be used to help break down and digest food. Medications to relieve pain and, where necessary, to treat any infection, may be prescribed.

> **SYMPTOMS OF PANCREATITIS**
>
> - A swollen, tender abdomen
> - Pain in the upper abdomen that radiates into the back
> - Nausea
> - Vomiting
> - Fever
> - A rapid heart rate
>
> If the condition becomes chronic, pancreatitis may cause weight loss because nutrients are not being absorbed, and it may lead to diabetes because a damaged pancreas cannot produce adequate insulin.

Gallstones can block the normal process of enzymes moving out of the pancreas into the small intestine, forcing the enzymes back into the pancreas, triggering irritation and inflammation. Where gallstones are related to pancreatitis, the stones and the gallbladder may be removed.

My Recommendations

There is good evidence that high triglycerides are associated with chronic pancreatitis. The best way to lower triglycerides is to eat less sugar, including fruit, and less starchy carbohydrates, such as white rice, potatoes, wheat, and other grain products. A diet high in vegetables, low in carbohydrates, and moderate in meat will significantly reduce risk and speed recovery from pancreatitis attacks.

Vegetables contain a number of enzymes that aid in digestion and reduce stress on the pancreas. Blenderized vegetables maximize the concentration of these enzymes (see the "Drink Your Veggies" chapter). In addition, vegetables contain a number of anti-inflammatory flavonoids that reduce the risk of inflammation damaging the pancreas.

Excitotoxins, described in more detail in the "Excitotoxins" chapter, increase inflammation in the pancreas and worsen the damage associated with pancreatitis. Glutamate, in MSG and other food additives, is a major excitotoxin that should be avoided. Because the pancreas contains a number of glutamate receptors, it is susceptible to damage from such additives. In addition to MSG, processed foods contain a number of disguised forms of glutamate additives, such as hydrolyzed protein, vegetable protein extracts and isolates, soy protein concentrates and isolates, autolyzed yeast, natural flavors, and carrageenan. In addition, some foods, such as mushrooms, cheeses, tomato sauces, broth, and stock, are naturally high in glutamate and should also be avoided.

Fluoride triggers inflammation and damages cells in the pancreas, as well as other tissues. It should always be avoided. Common sources include fluoridated drinking water, toothpaste, and mouthwash. Use filtered water and dental products without fluoride.

High iron levels can also damage the pancreas and lead to pancreatitis. For anyone with chronic or recurring pancreatitis, I recommend blood tests to measure total iron, transferrin, ferritin, and iron-binding capacity.

Natural Supplements
▶ N-Acetyl Cysteine (NAC)
NAC is a compound that safely increases cellular levels of glutathione, a major internal antioxidant in our bodies, which counteracts a degenerative process akin to internal rusting. It

also improves ongoing detoxification. Animal research shows that NAC powerfully inhibits damage caused by pancreatitis.

> ⬛ **What to do:** Take 500 to 750 mg, once a day with a full meal. It should never be taken on an empty stomach as it can cause severe stomach cramping. Should you develop stomach cramping, for quick relief, take two capsules of DGL plus, made by Pure Encapsulations. (DGL also relieves heartburn.)

▶ Curcumin

Curcumin is a powerful anti-inflammatory compound found in higher concentrations in the curry spice turmeric. Several studies indicate that the herbal extract can reduce damage caused by pancreatitis, in the pancreas and other organs. Curcumin also increases bile flow, thus reducing the risk of gallstones that can lead to pancreatitis.

> ⬛ **What to do:** Take 250 to 500 mg, three times a day, with meals. Use a highly absorbable form such as CurcumaSorb, made by Pure Encapsulations. Or, to improve absorption of powdered curcumin supplements, mix the powder contents of a capsule with a tablespoon of coconut or extra virgin olive oil. This can be messy.

▶ Apigenin

This is a natural flavonoid found in celery and parsley. A number of studies have shown that it quiets the cells that generate inflammation in the pancreas.

> ⬛ **What to do:** Take 100 mg (two capsules), three times a day, of Swanson's Apigenin. In severe cases, the dose can be increased to four capsules, three times a day.

▶ Resveratrol

This is a flavonoid that is concentrated in the skins of grapes and is found in varying quantities in red wine. One study found that it protects against damage to the pancreas. In addition, it protects the lungs and brain from damage that may be associated with pancreatitis. High doses should be taken with niacinamide, a B vitamin, as high resveratrol doses can lead to a shortage of cellular energy, and niacinamide prevents this.

> ➡ **What to do:** Take between 200 and 250 mg a day with food. If you take more than 300 mg daily, also take 500 mg of niacinamide daily.

▶ B Vitamins

The B vitamins are essential for our bodies to convert food into energy and help protect tissues and organs. A well-compounded formula should contain all the B vitamins in a form that is easily absorbed.

> ➡ **What to do:** Take one capsule a day of the Swanson Activated B-Complex High Bioavailability Formula, with or without food.

▶ Magnesium

The fourth most abundant mineral in the body, magnesium has powerful anti-inflammatory effects. Studies have shown that it reduces damage from pancreatitis and prevents disturbances in heart rhythm that can result from pancreatitis. Low magnesium levels dramatically increase one's risk of pancreatitis.

> ➡ **What to do:** For best absorption, take a slow-release form called Magnesium w/SRT, made by Jigsaw Health. Take one to two caplets, two or three times a day, with meals.

▶ Zinc

Many elderly people are quite deficient in this mineral. Zinc inhibits excitotoxicity and has anti-inflammatory properties. Experimental studies have shown that zinc reduces the damage caused by pancreatitis.

➡ **What to do:** The maintenance dose of zinc is 15 mg a day but severe deficiencies require higher amounts, based on blood tests of zinc levels.

▶ Buffered Vitamin C

Known as an antioxidant, vitamin C also reduces inflammation, regulates neurotransmitters, enhances immunity, stimulates cellular energy production, and has anticancer, antiviral, and antibacterial effects. Lypo-Spheric Vitamin C, made by LivOn Labs, is a highly absorbable, buffered form that is non-acidic and easy on the stomach. It comes in packets of gel that can be mixed with water or other liquids. High doses should be taken between meals, because when taken with food, vitamin C increases absorption of iron and can lead to iron overload.

➡ **What to do:** Take one packet (1,000 mg) of Lypo-Spheric Vitamin C, three times a day between meals.

▶ Mixed Tocopherols and Tocotrienols

In nature, vitamin E is a family of nutrients composed of four compounds called tocopherols and four compounds called tocotrienols. Together, they have strong anti-inflammatory effects, as well as antioxidant properties.

➡ **What to do:** Take 400 IU of mixed tocopherols and 50 mg of mixed tocotrienols, twice a day with meals.

▶ DHA

Short for docosahexaenoic acid, DHA is a component of omega-3 oils found in fish. It is one of the most abundant fats in membranes of all cells. Lab studies have shown that DHA can powerfully protect against tissue injury from pancreatitis. DHA is also found in certain types of algae.

➡ **What to do:** Take 1,000 to 2,000 mg a day of DHA, from fish oil or algae.

Ulcers

Also called peptic ulcers, these can develop in either the lining of the stomach or the upper part of the small intestine. In the stomach, they are called gastric ulcers, and in the small intestine, duodenal ulcers. In both cases, there is a sore (an erosion in the gut lining), which contains swollen and inflamed tissue that causes pain and discomfort. In a healthy digestive system, the special mucus-like secretions of the stomach and intestines protect against damage from stomach acid, but when there is an ulcer, the protection has broken down.

In the past it was thought that ulcers were caused by release of an excessive amount of stomach acid. Now it is known that most cases are caused by an infection. The most common cause is Helicobacter pylori, or H. pylori bacteria. However, many people who have these bacteria in their digestive tract do not get ulcers, and the reasons for this are not completely understood. It may have to do with the amount of stomach acid—those individuals with very low stomach acid are less affected by the H. pylori bacteria. This may explain why taking acid-lowering medications helps some people temporarily. There is also evidence that the species of the bacteria plays a major role—that is, some species of H. pylori are more likely to cause ulcerations than others. Chronic infections with H. pylori are also associated with gastric atrophy and a special form of stomach cancer.

Conventional Treatment

An ulcer is commonly diagnosed with an endoscopy, where a tiny camera mounted on a thin tube is inserted down the throat to look into the stomach, and a biopsy of the stomach lining may be done at the same time to check for H. pylori. Sometimes, a special type of x-ray is also used. Other ways to detect H. pylori include breath, blood, and stool tests. If H. pylori infection is present, antibiotics and other medications can treat it,

SYMPTOMS OF ULCERS

Some people who have an ulcer don't suffer pain, but these are common symptoms:

- Abdominal pain, especially between meals or at night
- An uncomfortable feeling of fullness
- Pain may last minutes or hours
- Food or antacids relieve pain
- Being unable to drink as much fluid as usual

and acid-suppressing drugs can help to relieve symptoms.

As well as causing pain and discomfort, ulcers that are untreated may bleed or even penetrate the wall of the stomach or intestine. Both events can cause severe complications or even death. At that point, ulcers can become very dangerous and require immediate medical or even surgical attention.

👍 My Recommendations

H. pylori infections of the stomach are a major player in stomach ulcers. However, there are other contributors and causes, such as prolonged stress, intense stress, alcohol abuse, smoking, and regular use of aspirin and other non-steroidal anti-inflammatory drugs (NSAIDs).

Recent studies have shown that certain foods can reduce the inflammation and damage to the stomach and intestinal lining, which causes the ulcer. The top therapeutic foods include strawberries, apples, and teas. It is important to choose organically grown fruits. In apples, the peel contains the most beneficial anti-ulcer compounds. One of the most effective compounds is chlorogenic acid, found in the highest concentrations in Macintosh apples.

🐰 Natural Supplements

Many natural plant extracts can significantly reduce ulcer-related damage and promote healing of the lining of the stomach and upper small intestine (the duodenum). Interestingly, these natural compounds work regardless of the cause of the ulcer—stress, alcohol abuse, NSAID use, or infection with H. pylori.

▶ Curcumin

Curcumin is a compound found in the spice turmeric in small amounts. Concentrated curcumin has a great number of beneficial effects, especially for protecting and healing the gastrointestinal tract. Studies have shown that curcumin possesses potent anti-ulcer activity and stimulates the healing of the damaged epithelial cells lining the stomach and intestine. It reduces inflammation and free radical damage, and inhibits destructive chemicals associated with ulcers.

➡ **What to do:** Take 250 mg, two to three times daily, ideally as a powder mixed with coconut oil. If it upsets your stomach, before taking the curcumin take DGL with water (see the "Heartburn" section for more details about DGL). Or, take it in a capsule that is specially formulated to be well absorbed: CurcumaSorb, made by Pure Encapsulations. One capsule contains 250 mg.

▶ Quercetin

Like curcumin, quercetin protects the lining of the stomach and intestines from damage, mainly by inhibiting inflammation and neutralizing free radicals—the main cause of ulcers. And like curcumin, quercetin is oil soluble. You can mix quercetin and curcumin together or you can purchase special high-absorption forms such as quercetin mixed with bromelain.

➡ **What to do:** Take 250 mg, three times daily with meals.

▶ Teas

A number of forms of tea have shown tremendous protection against peptic ulcers. In one study, researchers found that white, green, oolong, and black teas all had powerful anti-ulcer effects. At least two components in teas explain their protective effects—the presence of catechins and quercetin. I recommend using organic teas.

➡ **What to do:** Steep together one bag of white tea and one bag of oolong or black tea. Drink this tea three times a day. Drinking tea is a more pleasant way to take a health product than capsules or pills.

▶ Hesperidin

Found in high concentrations in oranges and orange juice, hesperidin is a powerful anti-inflammatory and antioxidant and has been shown to inhibit the growth of H. pylori.

➡ **What to do:** Take 250 mg, three times daily with meals.

▶ Ginger

A relative of curcumin, ginger has been shown to have powerful anti-ulcer properties. It is found in teas, other drinks, and in capsules. Fresh ginger can be grated or minced and added to rice, salads, salad dressings, vegetable side dishes, or mixed into drinks.

➡ **What to do:** Drink ginger tea or take 250 mg in a capsule with each meal. If more relief is needed, each dose can be increased up to 550 mg.

▶ DGL Plus

This is a combination of DGL (short for deglycyrrhizinated licorice) and other substances that coat and soothe the digestive tract, such as aloe vera, slippery elm, and marshmallow. It is made by Pure Encapsulations.

➡ **What to do:** Empty two capsules, mix with 4 ounces of water, and drink several times daily and before bedtime.

▶ Apigenin

This vegetable extract has been shown to reduce many of the serious complications of H. pylori infections of the stomach, such as atrophic gastritis, stomach cancer growth, and inhibits the growth of the bacteria.

➡ **What to do:** Take two 50 mg capsules of the Swanson's Apigenin three times a day.

▶ Optiberry

Optiberry is a supplement that contains a combination of blueberry, elderberry, strawberry, raspberry, and cranberry extracts. Studies have shown that it reduces gastric inflammation caused by H. pylori and reduces the growth of these organisms as well.

➡ **What to do:** Take two capsules three times a day on an empty stomach.

▶ Olive Leaf Extract and Olive Oil

Several compounds in extra virgin olive oil have been shown to suppress H. pylori bacteria, and olive leaf extract boosts cellular immune reactions against bacteria.

➡ **What to do:** One can take the olive leaf extract 500 mg per capsule at the same time as taking one tablespoon of extra virgin olive oil (use only high grade oil). Do this three times a day on an empty stomach.

▶ Probiotics

Studies have shown that several species of probiotic bacteria powerfully suppress the growth of H. pylori. These include mainly Lactobacillus salivarius and L. casei. Bifidobacterium also suppress its growth. L. lactis has the most potent activity against H. pylori, even at a low concentration. Some studies have shown that L. salivarius and L. rhmnosus eradicated H. pylori and reduced gastric inflammation as well.

➡ **What to do:** For those having active H. pylori infections I would recommend taking the 90 billion probiotic made by Garden-of Life once daily for 10 days and then once a week thereafter.

▶ Mastic Gum

This product is probably one of the most promoted for H. pylori treatment and there are reports of successful treatments. It is extracted as a tree resin (Pistacia lentiscus). One of the problems

I have found when using the product is that it can cause significant constipation in some people. Taking it with magnesium and high fiber intake will help with this problem.

➡ **What to do:** The recommended dose is two 500 mg capsules a day taken before breakfast.

CHAPTER 10

Liver

» Hepatitis B
» Hepatitis C
» Non-Alcoholic Liver Disease

Hepatitis B

This is a viral infection that may be acute or chronic and has been decreasing in the United States. According to the CDC, there are approximately 20,000 cases a year, a drop of 82 percent since 1991, when children began to be vaccinated against the disease. In fact, the United States had one of the lowest incidences of hepatitis B in the world before the vaccine. Chronic infections are now relatively rare. In fact, 90 percent of cases clear without any treatment within two years. However, hepatitis B is a serious problem globally, affecting about 240 million people and killing an estimated 786,000 per year, mostly in impoverished areas of the world.

The virus can be transmitted through bodily fluids, such as blood, semen, and vaginal fluids, but is not spread through food, water, breastfeeding, kissing, hugging, shaking hands, coughing, or sneezing. A pregnant women with hepatitis B can pass it on to her baby during childbirth.

Conventional Treatment

While antiviral medications are used for acute hepatitis B infections, they do not prevent recurrences. Rest and fluids, and sometimes hospitalization, are recommended. And once diagnosed, an individual should take precautions not to spread the disease.

For chronic infections, medications are not necessarily recommended because of side effects. However, the health of the liver should be monitored, alcohol should be avoided, and any prescription or over-the-counter drugs that may harm the liver should be avoided. In the United States, it's estimated that between 2,000 and 4,000 people die each year from liver disease related to hepatitis B. Cancer related to chronic hepatitis B is not a direct effect of the virus but secondary to long-term inflammation.

SYMPTOMS OF HEPATITIS B

Children under the age of 5 and about one-third of older children and adults do not have symptoms but over a period of years, or decades, are at a small risk of developing liver disease and liver failure, which can lead to disability or even death. Generally, symptoms appear between six weeks and six months after exposure to the virus, most often after about three months, and may include:

- Fatigue
- Loss of appetite
- Fever
- Stomach pain
- Dark urine
- Nausea
- Vomiting
- Joint pain
- Bowel movements that are clay-colored
- Jaundice (yellow skin or eyes)

My Recommendations

Experimental studies indicate that several plant extracts and nutrients, described below, can protect the liver in hepatitis B infections and eliminate the virus. Each works in a somewhat different way and a combination can improve the speed and extent of recovery.

Silymarin, from milk thistle, protects the liver. Curcumin and quercetin specifically kill the virus. Vitamin E has antiviral effects and lowers liver enzymes, which are a sign of damage to the liver. An extract from green or white tea (EGCG), and the teas themselves, prevent the hepatitis B virus from entering liver cells, thus preventing infection and re-infection, which can be a major problem.

Studies have shown that the hepatitis B virus can stop the immune system from defending itself, a mechanism called immune paralysis. Ellagic acid, extracted from plants such as pomegranates, can prevent this immune paralysis and make the virus susceptible to being killed by one's own immune system. Vitamin E also improves immunity to the hepatitis B virus.

Infected patients characteristically have low zinc and selenium levels, and increasing these protects the liver against damage. Vitamin C has powerful antiviral properties and reduces damage from inflammation that accompanies the disease.

Natural Supplements

▶ Curcumin

The herb kills the hepatitis B virus, reduces liver inflammation and free radicals, and improves bile flow. It also inhibits liver cancer.

> ➡ **What to do:** Take 500 mg, three times a day with meals. Use a product designed to be highly absorbable, such as CurcumaSorb, made by Pure Encapsulations, or mix a powdered form of curcumin with coconut or olive oil.

▶ Quercetin

A nutrient found in plants, quercetin has been shown to kill the virus, reduce inflammation, and help prevent cancer. It works best when combined with curcumin.

> ➡ **What to do:** Take 500 mg, three times a day with meals. The most absorbable form is Quercenase, made by Thorne

Research. Or, a powdered form of quercetin can be mixed with coconut or olive oil.

▶ Green Tea Extract (EGCG)

EGCG, short for epigallocatechin gallate, is the key therapeutic ingredient in green and white tea. It prevents the virus from entering liver cells and kills it.

➡ **What to do:** Take 100 mg, three times a day with meals. Teavigo is a standardized, caffeine-free extract in several brands, including a product made by Pure Encapsulations. Or, drink white tea, the richest natural source of EGCG.

▶ Ellagic Acid

Ellagic acid is a flavonoid, a therapeutic plant compound found in higher concentrations in pomegranates, raspberries, strawberries, and walnuts. It can prevent immune paralysis, which shuts off natural defenses against the hepatitis virus. By doing this, it makes the virus susceptible to being killed by one's immune system.

➡ **What to do:** Take 300 mg, three times a day with meals.

▶ Silymarin

An extract from milk thistle, silymarin can significantly lower elevated liver enzymes, a measure of liver damage in infected people, but does not kill the virus. It is best absorbed when combined with a fatty substance, as in Siliphos, made by Thorne Research. Otherwise, if you take a powdered extract, I suggest opening the capsule and mixing the contents with fish oil.

➡ **What to do:** Take 200 to 400 mg of any form, three times a day.

▶ Sulforaphane

Extracted from broccoli, sulforaphane improves liver detoxification, reduces inflammation, and has been shown to inhibit cancer.

▶ **What to do:** Take 400 mcg to 800 mcg, three times a day with meals. Swanson makes a good quality product with 400 mcg per capsule.

▶ Resveratrol

Found in high concentrations in grape skins, resveratrol has powerful anti-inflammatory and anticancer effects and raises levels of a major internal antioxidant in our bodies, glutathione.

▶ **What to do:** Take 200 mg daily, with a meal.

▶ Vitamin E

In nature, vitamin E has a combination of subtypes called mixed tocopherols, and this is the only form that should be used. It improves immunity to the virus, reduces inflammation, neutralizes free radicals, and has anticancer effects.

▶ **What to do:** Take 400 IU of mixed tocopherols, twice a day with meals.

▶ Vitamin C

Vitamin C is a powerful anti-inflammatory and antioxidant, and has anticancer properties. A buffered form called Lypo-Spheric Vitamin C, made by LivOn Labs, prevents acidity and is absorbed more effectively than regular vitamin C. It comes in packets of gel, each containing 1,000 mg of vitamin C.

▶ **What to do:** Mix two gel packets (2,000 mg) with water or juice and drink, three times a day. Higher doses can be used for more serious infections. Always take vitamin C on an empty stomach, as it increases iron absorption and taking it with food can lead to excess iron levels.

▶ Zinc Picolinate

Zinc levels are significantly low among people with hepatitis B, and with most other infections. Supplementing with zinc boosts the immune response to viral infections, and it also has antioxidant properties. Zinc picolinate is a specific form of the mineral.

➡ **What to do:** Take 50 mg a day for two weeks, then 50 mg twice a week thereafter. For severe infections, use an initial loading dose of 300 mg.

▸ Selenium (Selenomethionine)

The mineral plays a major role in immune function and is essential for important internal detoxification processes in our bodies. In addition, it has significant anticancer properties. Selenomethionine, available in several brands of supplements, is a form that is especially well absorbed.

➡ **What to do:** Take 400 mcg a day for three days and then reduce the dose to 200 mcg a day.

▸ Betatene

This is a mixture of a family of nutrients called carotenoids, which have antiviral properties. They boost immunity, protect the liver from damage, and promote detoxification. Betatene is a specific formula of carotenoids, made by Swanson.

➡ **What to do:** Take 25,000 IU (one capsule) twice a day.

Hepatitis C

There is no vaccine for hepatitis C, a viral infection that causes inflammation of the liver. It can be acute or chronic and, over the longer term, may lead to liver failure, liver cancer, and death. The virus is usually spread through blood, and less often through fluids exchanged during sex, but not through kissing, hugging, shaking hands, coughing, sneezing, food, or water. Its incidence is rising in the United States. Sharing of needles by drug addicts is a major source of the disease. Blood transfusions are another source, although in the

United States, donated blood is screened for the virus and other pathogens.

Most people who are infected have no symptoms, but may experience fatigue, loss of appetite, fever, stomach pain, dark urine, nausea, vomiting, joint pain, bowel movements that are clay-colored, or jaundice (yellow skin or eyes). This virus is more serious than the hepatitis B virus.

Conventional Treatment

It's estimated that about one in four people who are infected will clear the virus from their bodies without any treatment. For the rest, there are medications. Their effectiveness varies, depending upon the genetic variant of the virus, which can be determined with tests. With the right treatment, many cases can be cured.

Antiviral drugs can cause a number of complications, some serious, and treatment failures are common. Interferons, drugs designed to boost the immune system, are less successful than promotional efforts suggest and are accompanied by a number of significant and serious complications.

My Recommendations

Research with animals and several human studies have

WHO IS AT RISK?

People born between 1945 and 1965 are five times more likely to have hepatitis C, for reasons that are not really understood. The virus spreads chiefly through infected blood. People at risk include:

- Healthcare workers who suffer needlestick injuries

- Current or former drug users who have shared needles

- Kidney dialysis patients

- People infected with HIV

- Those who received blood transfusions or organ transplants in the United States before 1992, when blood banks began screening blood for the virus

- People who receive blood transfusions in countries where blood may be contaminated

- Babies born to mothers with hepatitis C

  Sharing razors or toothbrushes with an infected person or getting a tattoo or acupuncture treatment with an infected needle can also transmit the virus, but these are not common paths of infection.

found that various supplements reduce the duration of the infection and improve the extent of recovery. These include certain herbal extracts, vitamins, minerals, and healthy fats, which work in a variety of ways.

Curcumin fights the infection by inhibiting the entry of the virus into liver cells, inhibiting viral reproduction, and protecting liver cells from damage. Both curcumin and quercetin, a nutrient in plants, have been shown to specifically kill the hepatitis C virus. Silymarin, from milk thistle, inhibits entry of the virus into liver cells, reduces damage to the liver, and has improved hepatitis C cases that were difficult to treat and that were associated with severe liver scarring. An extract from green or white tea (EGCG), and the teas themselves, prevent the hepatitis C virus from entering liver cells, thus preventing infection and re-infection, which can be a major problem.

Studies have shown that the hepatitis C virus can stop the immune system from defending itself, a mechanism called immune paralysis. Ellagic acid, extracted from plants such as pomegranates, can prevent this immune paralysis and make the virus susceptible to being killed by one's own immune system. Vitamin E also improves immunity to the hepatitis C virus.

Infected patients characteristically have low zinc and selenium levels, and increasing these protects the liver against damage. Vitamin C has powerful antiviral properties and reduces damage from inflammation that accompanies the disease. Sulforaphane, from broccoli, has been shown to reduce the risk of liver cancer following chronic hepatitis C infection. In addition, branched chain amino acids—leucine, isoleucine, and valine—and fish oil, have been shown to promote liver healing.

In contrast, resveratrol, a generally beneficial ingredient in grape skins, is not recommended for hepatitis C (although it is helpful with hepatitis B). One study found that it significantly increased the replication of the virus.

🐇 Natural Supplements
▶ Curcumin

The herb kills the hepatitis B virus, and probably the hepatitis C virus as well, reduces liver inflammation and free radicals, and improves bile flow. It also inhibits liver cancer.

➡ **What to do:** Take 500 mg, three times a day with meals. Use a product designed to be highly absorbable, such as CurcumaSorb, made by Pure Encapsulations, or mix a powdered form of curcumin with coconut or olive oil.

▶ Quercetin

A nutrient found in plants, quercetin has been shown to kill the virus, reduce inflammation, and help prevent cancer. It works best when combined with curcumin.

➡ **What to do:** Take 500 mg, three times a day with meals. The most absorbable form is Quercenase, made by Thorne Research. Or, a powdered form of quercetin can be mixed with coconut or olive oil.

▶ Green Tea Extract (EGCG)

EGCG, short for epigallocatechin gallate, is the key therapeutic ingredient in green and white tea. It prevents the virus from entering liver cells and kills it.

➡ **What to do:** Take 100 mg, three times a day with meals. Teavigo is a standardized, caffeine-free extract in several brands, including a product made by Pure Encapsulations. Or, drink white tea, the richest natural source of EGCG.

▶ Ellagic Acid

Ellagic acid is a flavonoid, a therapeutic plant compound found in higher concentrations in pomegranates, raspberries, strawberries, and walnuts. It can prevent immune paralysis, which shuts off natural defenses against the hepatitis virus. By doing this, it makes the virus susceptible to being killed by one's immune system.

➡ **What to do:** Take 300 mg, three times a day with meals.

▶ Silymarin

An extract from milk thistle, silymarin can significantly lower elevated liver enzymes, a measure of liver damage in infected people, but does not kill the virus. It is best absorbed when combined with a fatty substance, as in Siliphos, made by Thorne Research. Otherwise, if you take a powdered extract, I suggest opening the capsule and mixing the contents with fish oil.

➡ **What to do:** Take 200 to 400 mg of either form, three times a day.

▶ Sulforaphane

Extracted from broccoli, sulforaphane improves liver detoxification, reduces inflammation, and has been shown to inhibit cancer.

➡ **What to do:** Take 400 mcg to 800 mcg, three times a day with meals. Swanson makes a good quality product with 400 mcg per capsule.

▶ Vitamin E

In nature, vitamin E has a combination of subtypes called mixed tocopherols, and this is the only form that should be used. It improves immunity to the virus, reduces inflammation, neutralizes free radicals, and has anticancer effects.

➡ **What to do:** Take 400 IU of mixed tocopherols, twice a day with meals.

▶ Vitamin C

Vitamin C is a powerful anti-inflammatory and antioxidant, and has anticancer properties. A buffered form called Lypo-Spheric Vitamin C, made by LivOn Labs, prevents acidity and is absorbed more effectively than regular vitamin C. It comes in packets of gel, each containing 1,000 mg of vitamin C.

➡ **What to do:** Mix two gel packets (2,000 mg) with water or juice and drink, three times a day. Higher doses can be used for more serious infections. Always take vitamin C on an empty stomach, as it increases iron absorption and taking it with food can lead to excess iron levels.

▶ Zinc Picolinate

Zinc levels are significantly low among people with hepatitis C, and with most other infections. Supplementing with zinc boosts the immune response to viral infections, and it also has antioxidant properties. Zinc picolinate is a specific form of the mineral.

➡ **What to do:** Take 50 mg a day for two weeks, then 50 mg twice a week thereafter. For severe infections, use an initial loading dose of 300 mg.

▶ Selenium (Selenomethionine)

The mineral plays a major role in immune function and is essential for important internal detoxification processes in our bodies. In addition, it has significant anticancer properties. Selenomethionine, available in several brands of supplements, is a form that is especially well absorbed.

➡ **What to do:** Take 400 mcg a day for three days and then reduce the dose to 200 mcg a day.

▶ Betatene

This is a mixture of a family of nutrients called carotenoids, which have antiviral properties. They boost immunity, protect the liver from damage, and promote detoxification. Betatene is a specific formula of carotenoids, made by Swanson.

➡ **What to do:** Take 25,000 IU (one capsule) twice a day.

▶ Branched Chain Amino Acids

Called BCAAs for short, these are three specific building blocks of protein: leucine, isoleucine, and valine. A number of studies have shown that they protect the liver and promote its healing.

➡ **What to do:** Take approximately 3 grams of a powder (between half and one scoop, depending on the product) mixed with water or juice, with a meal. Taking amino acids without food can trigger hypoglycemia—low blood sugar. For more severe liver injury, take the same amount up to three times a day.

▶ Fish Oil

Several studies have shown that the omega-3 fats in fish oil reduce liver inflammation and help protect liver cells from viral damage.

➡ **What to do:** Take one tablespoon daily of Liquid Fish Oil, made by Carlson. It should be kept in the refrigerator.

Non-Alcoholic Liver Disease

Often called the "silent" liver disease, the condition falls into two categories. Between 10 and 20 percent of Americans have non-alcoholic fatty liver disease, where fat accumulates in the liver but alcohol is not a contributing factor. A more serious condition, called non-alcoholic steatohepatitis, or NASH, affects up to 5 percent.

With NASH, fat in the liver is accompanied by inflammation, which damages the liver. As liver cells die, they are replaced by scar tissue, and if the scarring progresses far enough, it causes liver failure. However, even if the condition is simply fatty liver, without liver scarring, it is a sign of increased risk for heart disease and diabetes, which should be addressed.

Both types of fatty liver disease can be caused by alcohol abuse, but obesity and metabolic changes that precede diabetes are becoming more prevalent causes. NASH is the third most common reason for liver transplants, following alcohol abuse and hepatitis C. Non-alcoholic liver disease is also increasing in youth.

There is a strong connection between the increasing consumption of high fructose corn syrup (HFCS) and these liver disorders. A recent study found that when magnesium level is low, a high intake of HFCS dramatically increases the risk of metabolic damage that can lead to fatty liver disease. A great many processed foods contain the fructose sweetener.

SYMPTOMS OF FATTY LIVER DISEASE

In most cases, there are few if any symptoms of abnormal fat in the liver, but when it is accompanied by inflammation and damage to the liver, initial symptoms include fatigue, weakness, and weight loss. As cirrhosis–severe scarring and hardening of the liver–interferes with normal liver function to a greater degree, consequences may include:

- Intestinal bleeding
- Fluid retention
- Muscle wasting
- Liver failure
- Liver cancer

Conventional Treatment

Diet, exercise, weight loss, and avoidance of any unnecessary medications are today's treatment. There is no medication that corrects or reverses any type of fatty liver disease. If the condition progresses to a point of liver failure, a liver transplant is the only option.

My Recommendations

Since eating a diet rich in high fructose corn syrup is the leading cause of this liver disease, the most obvious thing is to stop eating such foods. Medications that stress the liver (warnings on labels should indicate this) should be avoided if possible. Switching to a diet mostly composed of vegetables, some meats, and lower amounts of carbohydrates would be most beneficial. Dietary fats do not cause fatty liver disease. However, omega-6 oils, such as corn, safflower, sunflower, peanut, and soybean oils, should be avoided, as these increase inflammation in the liver.

Certain herbs and nutrients are especially helpful in preventing a fatty liver disorder from progressing to the stages of liver scarring, hardening, and liver failure.

Natural Supplements

▶ Acetyl-L-Carnitine

A natural substance found in small quantities in meat, acetyl-L-carnitine dramatically improves the human body's internal processing of fats and reduces accumulation of harmful, inflammatory fats in the liver.

> ➡ **What to do:** Take 500 mg to 1,000 mg, two to three times a day with meals.

▶ R-Lipoic Acid

Like acetyl-L-carnitine, R-lipoic acid improves metabolism of fats and reduces accumulation of fats in the liver. A combination of the two nutrients is most effective for liver health.

> ➡ **What to do:** Take 100 mg to 300 mg, three times a day with meals.

▶ Curcumin

The herbal extract reduces liver inflammation, is an antioxidant, and improves bile flow, which reduces stress on the liver. It also inhibits liver cancer growth and invasion.

> ➡ **What to do:** Take 500 mg, three times a day with meals. Use a product designed to be highly absorbable, such as CurcumaSorb, made by Pure Encapsulations, or mix a powdered form of curcumin with coconut or olive oil.

▶ Quercetin

A nutrient found in plants, quercetin has been shown to inhibit liver inflammation and scarring. It is a very powerful anti-inflammatory, antioxidant, and anticancer nutrient which works best when combined with curcumin.

➤ **What to do:** Take 500 mg, three times a day with meals. The most absorbable form is Quercenase, made by Thorne Research. Or, a powdered form of quercetin can be mixed with coconut or olive oil.

▶ Silymarin

An extract from milk thistle, silymarin has been shown to protect liver cells, reduce inflammation, prevent fatty accumulation, and prevent liver scarring. It is best absorbed when combined with a fatty substance, as in Siliphos, made by Thorne Research. Otherwise, if you take a powdered extract, I suggest opening the capsule and mixing the contents with fish oil.

➤ **What to do:** Take 200 to 400 mg of either form, three times a day.

▶ Resveratrol

Found in high concentrations in grape skins, resveratrol has powerful anti-inflammatory and anticancer effects and raises levels of a major internal antioxidant in our bodies, glutathione.

➤ **What to do:** Take 200 mg daily, with a meal.

▶ Selenium (Selenomethionine)

The mineral plays a major role in immune function and is essential for important internal detoxification processes in our bodies. In addition, it has significant anticancer properties. Selenomethionine, available in several brands of supplements, is a form that is especially well absorbed.

➤ **What to do:** Take 400 mcg a day for three days and then reduce the dose to 200 mcg a day.

▶ Fish Oil

Several studies have shown that the omega-3 fats in fish oil reduce liver inflammation and help protect liver cells from damage by accumulated fats.

nat to do: Take one tablespoon daily of Liquid Fish Oil, made by Carlson. It should be kept in the refrigerator.

▶ **Magnesium Malate**

Magnesium has a number of beneficial effects. It reduces liver scarring and inflammation, improves blood flow and metabolism, and is an antioxidant. The most effective form is magnesium malate in a slow-release form, such as Magnesium w/SRT, made by Jigsaw Health.

➡ **What to do:** Take one slow-release tablet, three times a day with meals. For severe magnesium loss, it may be beneficial to increase each dose to two tablets.

CHAPTER 11

Cancer

Cancer Basics

There are more than a hundred types of cancer but they share a common characteristic. Unlike normal cells, which divide only a set number of times and then die, cancer cells just keep dividing. Ultimately, this create a mass of cells we call a tumor. Cancerous cells on the edges of the tumor can then invade surrounding healthy tissues, including the circulatory system, and can be carried to other parts of the body. This spreading of cancer, called metastasis, makes it deadly.

Localized cancers can usually be eliminated by surgery but once cancers spread, only 5 to 10 percent can be controlled long-term. There is a debate about whether cancers are ever cured as some return even decades after they appear to have been cured.

Stages of cancer are based on the degree to which they have spread. Stage 0 is a localized growth or tumor, which may or may not become full-blown cancer. Stage 1 is a localized cancerous growth and may be removed by surgery. Stages 2 and 3 are cancers that have invaded surrounding tissues to different degrees. Stage 4 is a cancer that has metastasized, meaning spread to distant parts of the body.

What Increases Cancer Risk?

According to the National Cancer Institute, only about 5 to 10 percent of cancers are caused by inherited genetic mutations. In the remaining 90 to 95 percent of cases, genetic mutations develop as a result of exposures to environmental toxins, such as tobacco smoke, radiation, other damaging substances, or due to lifestyle factors—all of which cause inflammation.

Smoking and obesity both increase risk for cancer. Abdominal obesity, in particular, is highly inflammatory. Age is also a factor, because as we get older, we become more inflamed and, as a result, cells are more likely to mutate and become cancerous. In addition, our immunity begins to falter as our cellular defense systems, which include detoxification mechanisms and antioxidant systems, start to decline.

Normally, we have a built-in immune surveillance system of special

A NEW SCIENTIFIC PERSPECTIVE

In the past, it was assumed that cancers arose from normal cells that became malignant. However, strong evidence now indicates that cancers arise from genetically damaged stem cells, not normal mature cells. These stem cells are like a child's bubble blower, generating an endless supply of primitive-looking cells that make up the bulk of the tumor. Inflammation, by generating massive amounts of free radicals, damages the genes of the stem cells and turns them into cancer stem cells. These cancer stem cells are resistant to most forms of chemotherapy and radiation treatment, which explains why so many cancers tend to recur after conventional treatments. In fact, most chemotherapy and radiation treatments increase the inflammation around the tumor and can make the tumor grow faster and become more aggressive.

cells that constantly survey our bodies, looking for cells that are damaged and at risk of becoming cancerous. When found, these potentially wayward cells are killed and removed. As we age, this surveillance system becomes less efficient.

All cells also contain special suicide genes, whose function is to kill cells that are damaged so badly that they risk becoming cancers. One example is the p53 gene. Approximately 50 percent of cancers are found to have mutations of this special gene and this prevents the cells from self-destructing, thus allowing the development of a cancer. Cancers with mutated p53 suicide genes are highly resistant to conventional treatments.

Most people are exposed to a number of cancer-causing agents and environmental risks. These include some dietary ingredients, toxic metals, nicotine and tobacco smoke, excess alcohol, unrelieved stress, and exposure to pesticides, herbicides, and fungicides. Some medications, such as statins, steroids, and TNF-alpha blockers, a class of drugs used to treat rheumatoid arthritis and other inflammatory diseases, increase risk by suppressing the immune system.

Conventional Treatment

Although an overall cure has not been found, most cancers are not a death sentence, especially if they are detected in an early stage, and can be destroyed with surgery, chemotherapy, or radiation. However, these all have serious side effects and are not always effective. Cancer cells can evade the action of one drug or can become resistant to all types of chemotherapy, a condition called multidrug resistance.

One innovative method involves testing the patient's tumor for sensitivity to a number of chemotherapy drugs, to determine the most effective drug. Another is seeking drugs that specifically target cancer stem cells, to potentially improve results and reduce side effects. So far, these are mostly in experimental stages and generally have a very high price tag.

👍 My Recommendations

Diet, such as the approach I suggest in "The Anti-Aging Pre-scription" chapter in this book, is the most important step for preventing cancer and aiding in its treatment, but there are many misconceptions about the diet-cancer link. For example, we hear a lot about fat and cancer, but not enough about the type of fat. These are the most important points:

Choose the right fats. I often refer to omega-6 fats, found in most vegetable oils, including corn, safflower, sunflower, peanut, canola, and soybean oils, as cancer fertilizers. These oils easily become oxidized, meaning they degrade, much like margarine turning rancid if it's left on the kitchen counter. And then they generate inflammation, which can damage genes. Never cook with these oils. Instead, use a saturated fat such as coconut oil, or extra virgin olive oil. Adding turmeric to oil reduces oxidation when cooking. Saturated animal fat does not promote growth of cancer cells but typically contains environmental toxins (such as pesticides and herbicides), less so if animals are raised according to organic standards.

Blenderize vegetables. Vegetables are the most important part of cancer prevention and treatment. To get the most benefit, I rec-ommend "blenderizing," meaning making a drink by blending raw vegetables with filtered water in a high-powered blender, such as a Vitamix. This unlocks many powerful anticancer compounds in the plants, which cannot otherwise be broken down and utilized by our digestive system. I also recommend eating a variety of raw and cooked vegetables, but never overlook blenderizing. It maxi-mizes nutrient absorption, preserves active enzymes, retains min-erals, and protects delicate, heat sensitive vitamins. For detailed instructions, see the "Drink Your Veggies" chapter.

Enlist top cancer fighters. Although all vegetables contain valuable nutrients, certain ones are especially rich in com-pounds that prevent and fight cancer. Leeks, onions, and garlic are powerful anticancer plants but are best eaten with meals, rather than in a vegetable drink. These rank high as cancer fighters and work well when blenderized:

- Cauliflower
- Cabbage
- Broccoli
- Brussels sprouts
- Kale
- Artichoke
- Bok choy
- Parsley
- Celery
- Leafy greens

Limit meats. The greatest dietary risk comes from eating too much heme iron, found in the highest levels in the blood of red meats. (Plants and egg yolks contain non-heme iron.) Heme iron is highly inflammatory and generates huge numbers of free radicals that are strongly linked to cancer development. Blood sausages and rare steaks are especially rich in heme iron and should be avoided. Eat no more than 4 ounces of meat, two to three times per week, and choose chicken over red meats. To reduce toxins found in conventionally raised meat, such as hormones and pesticides, aim for organic versions where possible, or choose meat from animals raised without hormones. Fish with low levels of mercury, typically smaller fish, are better choices.

Drink tea. Black, green, and white teas all contain powerful anticancer compounds. Drinking white or green tea can also reduce the cancer-causing effect of heme iron, by reducing its absorption. White tea is my favorite because it has the highest levels of beneficial nutrients and the lowest levels of fluoride. For variety, it can be mixed with herbal teas, such as pomegranate, blueberry, hibiscus, or chamomile teas, which also contain anticancer compounds. Drink at least two cups of white tea daily, hot or iced.

Spice things up. Turmeric, the curry spice, and ginger contain anticancer and anti-inflammatory substances. Fresh herbs, such as oregano, rosemary, thyme, sage, and others, generally contain a variety of antioxidants and anti-inflammatory substances, and all of these add flavor to food.

Avoid sugars and starches. Sugar is one of the primary fuels for cancer growth. Avoid high fructose corn syrup, other added sugars, sweetened drinks of any kind, fruit juices, and starchy carbohydrates, which are rapidly broken down into sugars. Choose high-fiber carbohydrates and eat only small amounts. Safe sweeteners include stevia and a product called Just Like Sugar®.

Go easy on fruit. Although fruit contains high levels of some anticancer compounds, it is also a source of natural sugars. For cancer prevention, berries, such as blueberries, strawberries, blackberries, and raspberries, can be included, as these are high in fiber and anticancer substances.

Some people eat a perfect diet, exercise regularly, and avoid toxins, yet still develop cancer and may even die as a result. The human being is an incredibly complex biological organism and there are many variables that determine our risk of developing and surviving cancer. For example, a person born with a weak immune system will face a higher risk than someone with a robust one. A strong family history of cancer or another disease that impairs resistance means more precautions need to be taken, including extra supplements to reduce cancer risk.

Natural Supplements

The supplements below provide basic nutritional support. Sections on breast, colon, lung, and prostate cancers provide more specific supplements for both prevention and treatment.

▶ Multivitamin/Mineral

Choose a product that does not contain iron but does contain 100 to 200 mcg of selenomethionine, a specific form of selenium that is effective against cancer.

➥ **What to do:** Take daily, per product directions.

▶ Vitamin E Succinate

This is a specific form of vitamin E shown to be superior to other forms of vitamin E as an anticancer nutrient.

➥ **What to do:** Take 400 IU, twice a day.

▶ Vitamin C

This is an essential vitamin for cancer protection. For easier digestion, it should be taken in a highly absorbable, buffered form that is not acidic, such as Lypo-Spheric Vitamin C, made by LivOn Labs, which comes in packets of gel which is mixed with water or other liquid. Each packet contains 1,000 mg of vitamin C.

➥ **What to do:** Take one packet (1,000 mg) of Lypo-Spheric Vitamin C, three times a day. Vitamin C should always be taken on an empty stomach, otherwise it increases iron absorption from foods and high doses can lead to iron overload.

▶ Beta Glucan

One of the most important weapons against cancer is the immune system. Beta glucan, technically called beta-1,3/1,6-glucan, stimulates anticancer immunity in cells, the most important natural defense against cancer. Beta glucan is an extract from the cell walls of baker's yeast.

➥ **What to do:** Take 500 mg, once a day for three days, and then every other day. Beta glucan should always be taken with water on an empty stomach. Do not eat for one hour after taking the supplement.

▶ **Hyperbaric Oxygen Therapy (HBOT)**

Cancer cells are highly vulnerable to oxygen, and several studies have found benefits from high oxygen levels, induced by hyperbaric oxygen therapy (HBOT). Such treatments reduce chemotherapy and radiation damage to healthy tissues and dramatically increase the sensitivity of the tumor to chemotherapy and radiation. HBOT also reduces inflammation that stimulates growth of cancers.

Breast Cancer

In the United States, about 12 percent of women will develop breast cancer at some point in life, according to the National Cancer Institute. But risk is much higher for women with specific, though rare, inherited genetic mutations.

Between 45 and 55 percent of those with a BRCA1 mutation, and 45 percent of those with a BRCA2 mutation, will develop breast cancer by age 70, and are more likely to develop the disease at a younger age. Together, BRCA1 and BRCA2 mutations account for 20 to 25 percent of hereditary breast cancers and 5 to 10 percent of all breast cancers. These genes control DNA repair and protect cells from genetic damage. Therefore, a mutation in either one increases risk.

The most common type of breast cancer, ductal carcinoma, begins in the ducts, which, in lactating women, carry milk to the nipples. The cancer can also form in the glands that make milk or in other breast tissue. When it becomes invasive, the cancer spreads from its origin point to the surrounding breast tissue and to lymphatic vessels and blood vessels. When it invades vessels, it can spread to distant areas of the body, especially the spine, brain, and liver.

As with all cancers, the central link is chronic inflammation in the area where the cancer develops. Studies have shown that women with high levels of inflammation markers in nipple secretions have a much greater risk of developing breast cancer. This inflammation can be from a number of causes, such as mastitis, fibrocystic disease, radiation exposure, exposure to pesticides and herbicides, and repeated trauma to the breast. Studies have shown that some pesticides accumulate in the ductal breast tissue so much that levels in the breast can be more than a hundred times higher than in the blood. An inflammatory diet plays a major role as well.

Women with poor DNA repair, poor detoxification systems, and elevated levels of inflammatory chemicals in the breast tissue have an increased risk of breast cancer. Couple this with a BRCA gene mutation and risk will be considerably greater.

> **GENETIC TESTING**
>
> The BRCA1 and BRCA2 mutations are relatively rare and, as a result, genetic testing for these is not recommended for all women. However, according to the National Cancer Institute, tests for these mutations should be done where family history includes:
>
> - Breast, ovarian, fallopian tube, or peritoneal cancer
> - Breast cancer diagnosed before age 50
> - Cancer in both breasts in the same woman
> - Both breast and ovarian cancers in either the same woman or the same family
> - Multiple breast cancers
> - Breast cancer in a male blood relative
> - Ashkenazi Jewish ethnicity

Conventional Treatment

Mammograms to detect abnormal tissue in breasts are recommended annually for women after age 40. And, if breasts are found to be dense, ultrasound is also recommended, as dense breasts can obscure smaller tumors on mammograms. However, many women are not informed about dense breast tissue and don't receive ultrasound screening, and this leads to missed cancers. If cancer is detected, surgery, chemotherapy, and/or radiation are the usual treatments.

The use of mammograms to detect breast cancer has come under serious scrutiny in medical literature, as several studies have shown an increased incidence of breast cancer in women who receive yearly screenings. Mammograms use radiation, which produces inflammation in the breast. This could increase risk for cancer, especially when combined with a poor diet, chronic inflammatory diseases, environmental toxins, and a BRCA gene mutation. There is also growing concern that far too many women are being diagnosed as having breast cancer when a tumor is actually a benign lesion. It is now accepted that as many as 80 percent of carcinoma in situ breast "cancers" are, in fact, benign tumors. When these tumors are misdiagnosed as breast cancer, women undergo unnecessary chemotherapy and radiation.

Metastatic breast cancers have a very low cure rate by conventional treatments—as low as 5 to 10 percent. Both radiation and chemotherapy carry a high complication rate and can induce other cancers later in life.

👍 My Recommendations

The most important weapon against breast cancer is the diet. A bad diet can cause chronic inflammation, impair detoxification systems in the liver and all cells, lower antioxidant defenses, weaken the immune system, and create conditions that increase the likelihood of cancer development, growth, and spread. Over time, a poor diet can also lead to frailty and chronic diseases, which make it more difficult to tolerate treatment, if cancer does develop. The most important dietary elements are described in the "Cancer Basics" section.

Exercise is also important and has been shown to reduce breast cancer risk. This can include brisk walking, resistance exercises, bike riding, or other moderately vigorous activity. Sedentary lifestyles increase the risk of frailty, chronic inflammation, depression, and poor immune function. Exercise should be done for at least 30 minutes, four to five times a week. Resistance exercise, which should work all the major muscles, is critical but often overlooked. It strengthens muscles, tendons, and ligaments, improves blood flow, improves lymphatic drainage and circulation, boosts our internal antioxidant function, reduces depression, increases energy levels, and improves the immune system.

Stress is a major source of inflammation and damaging free radicals. It can be mental or physical stress—especially if it involves a lack of sleep. Quality sleep is essential for good health and especially immune function. As we get older, we produce less of the sleep-inducing hormone melatonin, which has been shown to reduce cancer risk and can be taken as a supplement. If sleep is problematic, I prefer using the lowest dose of a sublingual melatonin supplement, around 0.5 mg, 30 minutes before bedtime.

Stress can be reduced in multiple ways, including: maintaining close family ties, socializing, having strong religious beliefs, attending your place of worship, listening to beautiful or inspiring music, watching enjoyable movies, or taking a vacation.

A healthy detoxification system strengthens resistance to cancers, as it cleanses the body of toxins, both from the environment and from the byproducts of one's metabolism. When detoxification is impaired, it is most often the result of a poor diet, which can be corrected. Detoxification takes place in the liver and in each cell in the body and can be improved by some supplements, such as quercetin, naringenin, and indole-3 carbinol, described below.

Natural Supplements
▶ Probiotics

Probiotic organisms in the colon play an important role in overall immunity and in protecting women from breast cancer. These friendly bacteria break down estrogen that is secreted by the liver into the colon and can reduce levels of harmful byproducts. And, probiotics improve the effectiveness of protective substances in flaxseed.

➧ **What to do:** Take a broad-spectrum probiotic, with a combination of beneficial bacteria and some prebiotics, which provide food for the beneficial organisms. One such product is Theralac, made by Master Supplements. Take one capsule of Theralac, at least once or twice a week. If you take a course of antibiotics, take two capsules, twice a day until the antibiotic is stopped, and then return to the lower dose. One can use the probiotics containing higher concentrations of organisms, such as the Garden of Life brand, containing 90 billion organisms of multiple species.

▶ Flaxseed Hull Lignans

Lignans are a therapeutic component of flaxseed. Bacteria in the colon convert compounds in the seed into powerful inhibitors of breast cancer. I prefer Flax Hull Lignans, made by Progressive Labs.

➧ **What to do:** Take one to two level tablespoons of Flax Hull Lignans, once or twice daily. Each dose contains 1.5 g of lignans. The powder can be added to a blenderized vegetable drink or mixed with water, juice, or goat's milk.

▶ DHA

Fish oil contains two key beneficial fats: EPA and DHA, and both reduce inflammation. However, DHA has the more powerful anticancer effects, for preventing and reducing growth of the cancer. DHA comes from algae, which is eaten by fish.

➧ **What to do:** Take 500 to 700 mg of DHA daily, in a fish oil or algae supplement.

▶ Curcumin

The herbal extract is a powerful inhibitor of breast cancer and protects the breast against damage from radiation in mammograms. In addition, it enhances the cancer-killing effects of chemotherapy and radiation treatments, while protecting the surrounding normal breast tissue. It also inhibits angiogenesis, which is the growth of blood vessels that feed a tumor, and cur-cumin can reverse multidrug resistance.

➡ **What to do:** For best absorption, use CurcumaSorb, made by Pure Encapsulations, which contains 250 mg per capsule. For protection, take 250 mg, twice a day with meals. High-er doses have been recommended for treatment of breast cancer—up to 1,000 mg, three to four times a day with food.

▶ Quercetin

Found in plants, quercetin inhibits the growth and spread of various types of breast cancers, and can reverse multidrug resis-tance. It is a powerful antioxidant and anti-inflammatory, espe-cially when taken with curcumin, and enhances the effectiveness of treatments while protecting healthy tissue. Quercenase, made by Thorne Research, is a well-absorbed form. If you use another brand, where capsules contain a powder, break them open and mix the powder with fish oil to increase absorption.

➡ **What to do:** For prevention, take 250 mg, two to three times a day with meals. Treatment requires higher doses, up to 1,000 mg, three times a day with meals.

▶ Apigenin and Naringenin

Studies have found that apigenin, a flavonoid found in higher concentrations in celery and parsley, is a superior anticancer agent. It powerfully suppresses inflammation, which precedes and promotes cancer, and inhibits development, growth, and spread of cancer. It works even better when combined with naringenin, also in the flavonoid family of nutrients, found in grapefruit and other citrus fruits.

➡ **What to do:** For prevention, take 50 to 100 mg of apigen-in, two to three times a day. During treatment, take up to 1,000 mg of apigenin, three times a day, with or without food. For prevention or treatment, take 500 mg of narin-genin, three times a day with meals.

▶ Luteolin

This is a flavonoid found in higher concentrations in celery, onion leaves, parsley, peppers, broccoli, cabbage, and carrots. Studies have shown it to be a potent cancer inhibitor by interfering with a number of cell-signaling pathways that support cancer cells. It also reduces the spread of cancer. I recommend the Luteolin Complex from Swanson.

➡ **What to do:** The most effective dose has not been precisely determined but a reasonable one would be 100 mg, three times a day, and up to 1,000 mg, three times a day. It can be taken with or without food.

▶ Silymarin

Studies have shown that this extract of the milk thistle plant increases the cancer-killing power of chemotherapy agents, inhibits cancer invasion, increases self-destruction (apoptosis) of breast cancer cells, and is highly effective against estrogen-negative breast cancer, the most deadly form. Its ability to enhance liver function, especially detoxification, is of major importance in breast cancer treatment.

➡ **What to do:** Silymarin is poorly absorbed as a powder. To improve absorption, mix the contents of capsules with a tablespoon of fish oil or extra virgin olive oil. Or, use Siliphos, made by Thorne Research, which is a well absorbed form. Take 200 mg, twice a day with food.

▶ Indole-3-carbinol (I3C) or DIM

Indole-3-carbinol, or I3C for short, is found in high concentrations in cruciferous vegetables, especially Brussels sprouts and broccoli. DIM (short for diindolylmethane) is another form of the compound. In the human body, either form can be converted to the other. Both forms are equally effective against cancers of the breast and prostate. Indole-3-carbinol has been shown to inhibit spread of breast cancer to bones, a common site of

metastasis. It also enhances the effectiveness of several chemotherapy drugs used to treat breast cancer, and has strong anticancer activity against triple negative breast cancer, one of the
most deadly types.

➡ **What to do:** Use either indole-3-carbinol or DIM. I suggest taking 100 mg of DIM, three times a day with meals,
in DIM-Pro 100, made by Pure Encapsulations, as it has
been tested in studies. Or, take 400 mg of indole-3-carbi-
nol, three times a day with meals.

▶ Berberine

Berberine is a powerful and versatile anticancer agent with a
wide margin of safety. Several studies have shown that it inhibits
breast cancer by a number of mechanisms. In addition, it reduces the harmful effects of chemotherapy on normal tissues and
organs and is particularly effective against doxorubicin toxicity
on the heart, a major complication of the drug. Berberine also
makes breast cancer cells—especially breast cancer stem cells—
more sensitive to the killing effects of radiation treatment.

➡ **What to do:** Take 400 mg, three times a day with meals.

▶ Protease Enzymes

Another innovative treatment is the use of protein-dissolving
enzymes called proteases. Cancer cells protect themselves from
being destroyed by the immune system by cloaking themselves
with a layer of antibodies called antibody complexes. The protease enzymes dissolve these cloaking antibodies, exposing the
cancer cells to destruction by the body's immune cells. The enzymes have to be taken on an empty stomach, because otherwise, they are not absorbed.

➡ **What to do:** Wobenzym N is a product with a combination of protease enzymes that has been successfully used
for many years. The usual dose is six tablets, three times a
day between meals.

▶ Vitamin D3

This is the active form of vitamin D. Studies have shown that women with low vitamin D3 levels have a higher incidence of breast cancer than those with normal or higher levels. Improving anti-tumor immunity is one of its benefits.

➡ **What to do:** Get a vitamin D blood test before taking supplements. The normal range is between 35 and 100 ng/ml. Above 100 ng/ml, we see immune suppression. Take the amount recommended after a test. Get blood levels re-checked after three weeks of supplementation, and less frequently after that. A maintenance dose is 2,000 IU a day but with severe deficiencies, much higher doses are required.

▶ Hyperbaric Oxygen Therapy (HBOT)

Hyperbaric oxygen therapy with 100 percent oxygen can be of benefit for a number of cancers, including breast cancer. Cancer thrives in a low-oxygen environment. High levels of oxygen can kill cancer cells, reduce growth of blood vessels that feed tumors, enhance the effectiveness of radiation and chemotherapy treatments, and reduce harmful effects of such treatments on healthy tissues and organs. HBOT also inhibits inflammation, a major stimulus of cancer growth and invasion.

Colon Cancer

The third most common cancer among American men and women, colorectal cancer is found in the colon or the rectum, both part of the large intestine—the lower part of the digestive system. The incidence increases significantly after age 50, much more among people with chronic inflammatory bowel diseases. Other triggers of inflammation, which also increase risk, include unresolved gluten sensitivity or an imbalance of gut bacteria, which normally help prevent inflammation in the lining of the colon. A deficiency of beneficial bacteria and/or an overabundance of harmful bacteria can lead to a chronically inflamed colon and a significantly greater risk of colon cancer.

The most common early signs include a change in bowel habits with diarrhea (especially if bloody), constipation, alteration of the two, and rectal bleeding. Anemia with low hemoglobin levels is sometimes a sign of colon cancer.

If diagnosed early, the cure rate is between 80 and 90 percent, but because many cases are not detected right away, the overall cure rate is about 50 percent. If this cancer metastasizes, the cure rate is only 5 to 10 percent. Some colon cancers are slower growing while others are quite aggressive and metastasize quickly.

Colonoscopies and tests for blood in the stool are common diagnostic tools for detecting abnormalities that may develop into the cancer. Polyps, benign growths in the colon, may be an early sign, but not all polyps become cancerous.

RISK FOR COLON CANCER

The odds of colon cancer increase with:
- Age over 50
- Colon polyps
- Crohn's disease
- Ulcerative colitis
- Other types of chronic bowel inflammation
- Celiac disease
- Family history of colon polyps
- Family history of colon cancer

Blood in the stool or changes in bowel habits may indicate colon cancer development, but may also be due to other, unrelated factors.

Conventional Treatment

If the cancer is localized and has not spread, surgery alone may remove it all, with no further treatment. In the case of a cancerous polyp with no penetration into deeper layers, only the polyp may need to be removed. But if the cancer has spread into the deeper layers of the colon, part of the colon, and sometimes adjoining tissue, may also be removed. Intra-abdominal lymph nodes are examined to make sure the tumor has not spread.

Chemotherapy or radiation may also be used if doctors are not certain that all the cancerous tissue has been taken out, or if it has penetrated the bowel wall and traveled to the local lymph nodes. When patients are not strong enough to withstand surgery, chemotherapy or radiation is sometimes the only treatment.

👍 My Recommendations

The most important weapon against colon cancer is the diet. A bad diet can cause chronic inflammation, impair normal detoxification systems in the liver and all cells, lower antioxidant defenses, weaken the immune system, and create conditions that increase the likelihood of cancer development and spread. Over time, a poor diet can also lead to frailty and chronic diseases, which make it more difficult to tolerate treatment.

The most important dietary elements are described in the "Cancer Basics" section, but there are some additional ones for colon cancer prevention or recovery. One's diet should consist mostly of cruciferous vegetables and other anticancer plants, such as onions, garlic, greens, spinach, celery, and parsley. Blenderized vegetables are best. Breads and other foods containing gluten should be eaten only in limited amounts, and if one is gluten sensitive or already has a tumor, they should be avoided altogether.

For colon health, it's vital to drink liquids throughout the day to improve lymphatic drainage and circulation in tiny microvessels that deliver blood to tissues. White and green teas are the best beverages because they contain powerful inhibitors of colon cancer and reduce absorption of harmful heme iron from meat. Glutamate, as found in MSG and other excitotoxin additives, should be avoided because it can stimulate the growth and invasion of colon cancers. For different ways in which it is disguised on food labels, see the chapter "Excitotoxins."

Exercise is also important and has been shown to reduce colon cancer risk. It can include brisk walking, resistance exercises, bike riding, or other moderately vigorous activity.

Sedentary lifestyles increase the risk of frailty, chronic inflammation, depression, and poor immune function. Exercise for at least 30 minutes, four to five times a week. Resistance exercise, which should work all the major muscles, is critical but often overlooked. It strengthens muscles, tendons, and ligaments, improves blood flow, improves lymphatic drainage and circulation, boosts internal antioxidant systems, reduces depression, increases energy levels, and improves the immune system.

Stress is a major source of inflammation and damaging free radicals. It can be mental or physical stress—especially if it involves a lack of sleep. Quality sleep is essential for good health and especially immune function. As we get older, we produce less of the sleep-inducing hormone melatonin, which has been shown to reduce cancer risk. It can be taken as a supplement. If sleep is problematic, I prefer using the lowest dose of a sublingual melatonin supplement, around 0.5 mg, 30 minutes before bedtime.

Stress can be reduced in multiple ways, including: maintaining close family ties, socializing, having strong religious beliefs, attending your place of worship, listening to beautiful or inspiring music, watching enjoyable movies, or taking a vacation.

A healthy detoxification system strengthens resistance to cancers, as it cleanses the body of toxins, both from the environment and from the byproducts of one's metabolism. When detoxification is impaired, it is most often the result of a poor diet, which can be corrected. Detoxification takes place in the liver and in each cell in the body and can be improved by some supplements, such as quercetin and naringenin, described below.

Natural Supplements
▶ Flaxseed Hull Lignans
Lignans are a therapeutic component of flaxseed. Bacteria in the colon convert compounds in the seed into powerful inhibitors of colon cancer. I prefer Flax Hull Lignans, made by Progressive Labs.

➧ **What to do:** Take one to two level tablespoons of Flax Hull Lignans, once or twice daily. Each dose contains 1.5 g of lignans. The powder can be added to a blenderized vegetable drink or mixed with water, juice, or goat's milk.

▶ Probiotics

Probiotic organisms in the colon play an important role in protecting against colon cancer. In addition to regulating inflammation in the colon, they turn certain compounds in flaxseed into powerful cancer inhibitors. And, they produce butyric acid (see below).

➧ **What to do:** Eat fermented foods or take a broad-spectrum probiotic with a combination of beneficial bacteria, such as Theralac, made by Master Supplements.

▶ Butyric Acid

A byproduct of fiber digestion, butyric acid slows the growth and invasion of colon cancers. People with low levels of butyric acid in the colon have a significantly higher risk of developing the cancer. Butyri Plex, made by American Biologics, is a good quality supplement.

➧ **What to do:** Take one capsule (750 mg) of Butyri Plex, three times a day with meals. To increase its effectiveness in targeting and killing colon cancer cells, take it with Teavigo and DHA, described below.

▶ Teavigo

A standardized extract from green tea, Teavigo contains exceptionally high concentrations of EGCG, the therapeutic ingredient in the tea. Studies have shown that it powerfully inhibits colon cancer in multiple ways. In animal studies, EGCG prevented colon cancer from metastasizing to the liver, one of the most frequently affected sites. White and green teas are high in EGCG.

▶ **What to do:** For prevention, take one capsule of Teavigo (100 mg) daily with a meal. During treatment, take one capsule, three times a day with meals. Anyone who has documented liver damage or takes medications that damage the liver should not take Teavigo or any other EGCG supplement.

▶ DHA

Fish oil contains two key beneficial fats: EPA and DHA, and both reduce inflammation. However, DHA has the more powerful anticancer effects for preventing and reducing growth of the cancer. DHA comes from algae, which is eaten by fish.

▶ **What to do:** Take 500 to 700 mg of DHA daily, in a fish oil or algae supplement.

▶ Curcumin

The herbal extract is a powerful inhibitor of colon cancer and can protect other organs and tissues in the abdomen from damage during radiation treatments. In addition, it enhances the cancer-killing effects of chemotherapy and radiation treatments, inhibits angiogenesis, which is the growth of blood vessels that feed a tumor, and can reverse multidrug resistance.

▶ **What to do:** For best absorption, use CurcumaSorb, made by Pure Encapsulations, which contains 250 mg per capsule. For protection, take 250 mg, twice a day with meals. Higher doses have been recommended for treatment of colon cancers—up to 1,000 mg, three to four times a day with food.

▶ Quercetin

Found in plants, quercetin inhibits the growth and spread of various cancers and can reverse multidrug resistance. It is a powerful antioxidant and anti-inflammatory, especially when taken with curcumin, and enhances the effectiveness of treatment while protecting healthy tissues. Quercenase, made by Thorne Research, is a well-absorbed form. If you use another brand, where capsules contain a powder, break them open and mix the powder with fish oil or olive oil to increase absorption.

➡ **What to do:** For prevention, take 250 mg, two to three times a day with meals. Treatment requires higher doses, up to 1,000 mg, three times a day with meals.

▶ Silymarin

Studies have shown that this extract of the milk thistle plant increases the cancer-killing power of chemotherapy agents, inhibits cancer invasion, increases self-destruction (apoptosis) of colon cancer cells, and inhibits the growth of colon cancer stem cells. Its ability to enhance liver function, especially detoxification, is of major importance in colon cancer treatment.

➡ **What to do:** Silymarin is poorly absorbed as a powder. To improve absorption, mix the contents of capsules with a tablespoon of fish oil or extra virgin olive oil. Or, use Siliphos, made by Thorne Research, which is a well absorbed form. Take 200 mg, twice a day with food.

▶ Apigenin and Naringenin

Studies have found that apigenin, a flavonoid found in higher concentrations in celery and parsley, is a superior anti-cancer agent. It powerfully suppresses inflammation and inhibits development, growth, and spread of cancer. It works even better when combined with naringenin, also in the flavonoid family of nutrients, found in grapefruit and other citrus fruits.

➡ **What to do:** For prevention, take 50 to 100 mg of apigenin, two to three times a day. During treatment, take up to 1,000 mg of apigenin, three times a day, with or without food. For prevention or treatment, take 500 mg of narin-genin, three times a day with meals.

▶ Luteolin

This is a flavonoid found in higher concentrations in celery, onion leaves, parsley, peppers, broccoli, cabbage, and carrots. Studies have shown it to be a potent cancer inhibitor by inter-fering with a number of cell-signaling pathways that support cancer cells. It also reduces the spread of cancer. I recommend the Luteolin Complex from Swanson.

➡ **What to do:** The most effective dose has not been pre-cisely determined but a reasonable one would be 100 mg, three times a day, and up to 1,000 mg, three times a day. It can be taken with or without food.

▶ Vitamin D3

This is the active form of vitamin D. Studies have shown that people with low vitamin D3 levels have a much higher incidence of colorectal cancer than those with normal or higher levels. Im-proving anti-tumor immunity is one of its benefits.

➡ **What to do:** Get a vitamin D blood test before taking sup-plements. The normal range is between 35 and 100 ng/ml. Above 100 ng/ml, we see immune suppression. Take the amount recommended after a test. Get blood levels re-checked after three weeks of supplementation, and less fre-quently after that. A maintenance dose is 2,000 IU a day but with severe deficiencies, much higher doses are required.

▶ Ellagic Acid

A therapeutic substance in various plant foods, ellagic acid is found in higher concentrations in raspberries, pomegranates, strawberries, and walnuts. It enhances the immune system and is a potent cancer inhibitor.

➡ **What to do:** Take 300 mg, three times a day with meals.

▶ Berberine

This natural plant compound inhibits cancer growth, cancer stem cells, and invasion of the bowel wall, reducing the risk of colon cancer metastasis. In people with a family history of colon polyps, it inhibits the growth of polyps.

> ➡ **What to do:** Take 500 mg, three times a day with meals. Berberine-500, made by Thorne Research, is a good quality product. One caution: In people with a history of reactive hypoglycemia, berberine can cause headaches.

▶ Hyperbaric Oxygen Therapy (HBOT)

Hyperbaric oxygen therapy with 100 percent oxygen has enhanced chemotherapy or radiation treatment when either of these were given immediately after the HBOT treatment. The effect was more pronounced on radiation treatment. Only a limited number of studies have been done and show that HBOT treatment alone did not enhance tumor killing but may have reduced tumor invasion by inhibiting angiogenesis, meaning the growth of blood vessels that feed a tumor.

Lung Cancer

Lung cancer accounts for about 13 percent of all cancers in the United States but 27 percent of all cancer deaths, according to the American Cancer Society. Although there are nearly a half-million Americans who had lung cancer and are alive today, the prognosis is generally not good. It's estimated that roughly 220,000 new cases and 158,000 deaths occur each year.

Survival depends largely upon the stage at which the cancer is diagnosed, but screening raises questions. In the past, yearly chest x-rays were recommended but then dropped after studies demonstrated no real benefits and a real danger of repeated radiation exposure. Detection of small abnormalities requires

CT scans, which expose the person to large amounts of radiation. In addition, routine scanning can detect suspicious lesions that require biopsy, which can have serious complications. In many cases, early-stage lung cancer is detected accidentally during testing for other health conditions.

There are two major types of lung cancer: adenocarcinoma and squamous cell cancer—the most common form and the one most closely associated with smoking. Before women smoked, they rarely developed lung cancer, but once they began to smoke in massive numbers, incidence of lung cancer among women increased, matching that of men. As the rate of smoking has declined, the overall incidence of lung cancer has fallen, yet there is an increase in lung cancer not related to smoking.

> **WHO SHOULD BE SCREENED?**
>
> The American Cancer Society recommends screening with low-dose CT scans only for people who meet all these criteria:
>
> - Age 55 to 74
> - Are in fairly good health
> - Have smoked at least the equivalent of a pack a day for 30 years
> - Still smoke or quit smoking within the last 15 years

Conventional Treatment

Treatment depends upon the stage at which a lung cancer is diagnosed. Most people have no symptoms and are not diagnosed until they have progressed beyond the point of cure. People who have symptoms such as coughing, wheezing, shortness of breath, weakness, feeling tired, coughing up blood, or persistant respiratory infections should see their doctor, as these could be signs of many conditions.

Treatment may include surgery, radiation, chemotherapy, and other drugs. In some cases, genetic testing and culture testing may be done to identify the most effective drugs. Since most cases are metastatic at the time of diagnosis, the prognosis with conventional treatment is dismal.

👍 My Recommendations

The most important weapon against lung cancer is the diet. A bad diet can cause chronic inflammation, impair detoxification systems in the liver and all cells, lower antioxidant defenses, weaken the immune system, and create conditions that increase the likelihood of cancer development, growth, and spread. Over time, a poor diet can also lead to frailty and chronic diseases, which make it more difficult to tolerate treatment if cancer does develop.

The most important dietary elements are described in the "Cancer Basics" section, but there are some additional ones for lung cancer prevention or treatment. Diet should consist mostly of cruciferous vegetables, as these inhibit lung cancer. Other good anticancer plant foods include onions, garlic, greens, spinach, celery, and parsley. Blenderized vegetables are best. Breads and other foods containing gluten should be eaten only in limited amounts and should be avoided altogether if one is gluten-sensitive or already has a tumor.

For healthy lungs, it's vital to drink liquids throughout the day to improve lymphatic drainage and circulation in tiny microvessels that deliver blood to tissues. White and green teas are the best beverages because they contain powerful inhibitors of lung cancer and reduce absorption of harmful heme iron from meat. Glutamate, as found in MSG and other excitotoxin additives, should be avoided because it can stimulate the growth and invasion of lung and other cancers. For different ways in which it is disguised on food labels, see the chapter "Excitotoxins."

Smoking and the use of nicotine patches should be avoided, as nicotine lowers immunity and thus increases cancer risk. Also avoid exposure to other toxins, including pesticides, herbicides, industrial chemicals, automobile exhaust fumes, radon gases, and toxic metals such as aluminum, lead, mercury, arsenic, cadmium, and manganese.

Exercise is also important and has been shown to reduce the risk of most cancers. This can include brisk walking, resistance exercises, bike riding, or other moderately vigorous activity. Sedentary lifestyles increase the risk of frailty, chronic inflammation, depression, and poor immune function. Exercise at least for 30 minutes, four to five times a week. Resistance exercise, which should work all the major muscles, is critical but often overlooked. It strengthens muscles, tendons, and ligaments, improves blood flow, improves lymphatic drainage and circulation, boosts our internal antioxidant function, reduces depression, increases energy levels, and improves the immune system.

Stress is a major source of inflammation and damaging free radicals. It can be mental or physical stress—especially if it involves a lack of sleep. Quality sleep is essential for good health and especially immune function. As we get older, we produce less of the sleep-inducing hormone melatonin, which has been shown to reduce cancer risk and can be taken as a supplement. If sleep is problematic, I prefer using the lowest dose of a sublingual melatonin supplement, around 0.5 mg, 30 minutes before bedtime.

Stress can be reduced in multiple ways, including: maintaining close family ties, socializing, having strong religious beliefs, attending your place of worship, listening to beautiful or inspiring music, watching enjoyable movies, or taking a vacation.

A healthy detoxification system strengthens resistance to cancers, as it cleanses the body of toxins, both from the environment and from the byproducts of one's metabolism. When detoxification is impaired, it is most often the result of a poor diet, which can be corrected. Detoxification takes place in the liver and in each cell in the body and can be improved by some supplements, such as quercetin and naringenin, described below.

Natural Supplements

▶ DHA

Fish oil contains two key beneficial fats: EPA and DHA, and both reduce inflammation. However, DHA has the more powerful anticancer effects for preventing and reducing growth of the cancer. DHA comes from algae, which is eaten by fish.

➡ **What to do:** Take 500 to 700 mg of DHA daily, in a fish oil or algae supplement.

▶ Curcumin

The herbal extract is a powerful inhibitor of lung cancer and can protect healthy organs from damage during radiation treatments. In addition, it enhances the cancer-killing effects of chemotherapy and radiation treatments, inhibits angiogenesis, which is the growth of blood vessels that feed a tumor, and can reverse multidrug resistance. Studies also indicate that curcumin can reduce the invasiveness and metastatic spread of lung cancer.

➡ **What to do:** For best absorption, use CurcumaSorb, made by Pure Encapsulations, which contains 250 mg per capsule. For protection, take 250 mg, twice a day with meals. Higher doses have been recommended for treatment of lung cancers—up to 1,000 mg, three to four times a day with food.

▶ Quercetin

Found in plants, quercetin inhibits the growth and spread of various cancers, including lung cancer, and can reverse multidrug resistance. It is a powerful antioxidant and anti-inflammatory, especially when taken with curcumin, and enhances the effectiveness of treatment while protecting healthy tissues. Quercenase, made by Thorne Research, is a well-absorbed form. If you use another brand, where capsules contain a powder, break them open and mix the powder with fish oil or olive oil to increase absorption.

➡ **What to do:** For prevention, take 250 mg, two to three times a day with meals. Treatment requires higher doses, up to 1,000 mg, three times a day with meals.

▶ Silymarin

Studies have shown that this extract of the milk thistle plant increases the cancer-killing power of chemotherapy agents, inhibits cancer invasion, increases self-destruction (apoptosis) of lung cancer cells, and inhibits the growth of lung cancer stem cells. Its ability to enhance liver function, especially detoxification, is of major importance in lung cancer treatment.

➡ **What to do:** Silymarin is poorly absorbed as a powder. To improve absorption, mix the contents of capsules with a tablespoon of fish oil or extra virgin olive oil. Or, use Siliphos, made by Thorne Research, which is a well absorbed form. Take 200 mg, twice a day with food.

▶ Apigenin and Naringenin

Studies have found that apigenin, a flavonoid found in higher concentrations in celery and parsley, is a superior anticancer agent. It powerfully suppresses inflammation and inhibits development, growth, and spread of cancer. It works even better when combined with naringenin, also in the flavonoid family of nutrients, found in grapefruit and other citrus fruits.

➡ **What to do:** For prevention, take 50 to 100 mg of apigenin, two to three times a day. During treatment, take up to 1,000 mg of apigenin, three times a day, with or without food. For prevention or treatment, take 500 mg of naringenin, three times a day with meals.

▶ Luteolin

This is a flavonoid found in higher concentrations in celery, onion leaves, parsley, peppers, broccoli, cabbage, and carrots. Studies have shown it to be a potent cancer inhibitor by interfering with a number of cell-signaling pathways that support cancer cells. It is also a powerful inhibitor of tumor invasion and sensitizes lung cancer cells to radiation treatments, while protecting surrounding healthy cells. I recommend the Luteolin Complex from Swanson.

➡ **What to do:** The most effective dose has not been precisely determined but a reasonable one would be 100 mg, three times a day, and up to 1,000 mg, three times a day. It can be taken with or without food.

▶ Resveratrol

In lab studies, resveratrol has powerfully suppressed the growth of lung cancers in a dose that would be equivalent to 210 mg in a human. It also inhibits spread of the cancer, enhances effectiveness of chemotherapy, and helps to prevent multidrug resistance. Animal research found that a combination of curcumin and resveratrol is even more effective.

➡ **What to do:** The most effective dose appears to be between 250 and 500 mg, taken once a day with a meal.

▶ Teavigo

A standardized extract from green tea, Teavigo contains exceptionally high concentrations of EGCG, the therapeutic ingredient in the tea. Studies have shown that it powerfully inhibits lung cancer development and spread, as well as enhancing chemotherapy effectiveness and reducing radiation damage to the esophagus, which frequently occurs with radiation treatments for lung cancer. EGCG is especially powerful at inhibiting some of the most invasive lung cancers and those that have become resistant to chemotherapy drugs. In addition, it can reduce muscle loss, which is commonly seen with lung cancer.

➡ **What to do:** For prevention, take one capsule of Teavigo (100 mg) daily with a meal. During treatment, take one capsule, three times a day with meals. Anyone who has documented liver damage or takes medications that damage the liver should not take Teavigo or any other EGCG supplement.

▶ Berberine

This natural plant compound inhibits inflammation, growth of cancer cells and stem cells, and invasion of lung cancer into surrounding healthy tissues. In addition, it increases cancer-cell death from chemotherapy.

➡ **What to do:** Take 500 mg, three times a day with meals. Berberine-500, made by Thorne Research, is a good quality product. One caution: in people with a history of reactive hypoglycemia, berberine can cause headaches.

▶ Hyperbaric Oxygen Therapy (HBOT)

Few studies have been done using HBOT for lung cancers, but one clinical study that combined photodynamic therapy with HBOT did see significant improvement in the patient's symptoms. More study is needed to determine if HBOT is useful in treating lung cancer patients.

Prostate Cancer

Most often, prostate cancer grows very slowly and many cases are not deadly. It generally develops in prostate gland cells that make fluid and is most common among men over the age of 65. It varies from a very benign form, which grows very slowly and rarely spreads, to very aggressive tumors that invade early and spread throughout the body. By age 70, around 70 percent of men have cancer cells in their prostate gland, yet most will never develop full blown prostate cancer.

In the past, the prostate specific antigen (PSA) test was thought to be of value as a screening tool, but most cases of elevated PSA are related to benign conditions. However, rapid elevation in PSA is a warning sign.

The cancer is more common, more aggressive, and more deadly among men who are African American, possibly because

WHAT INCREASES RISK?

Six in ten cases of prostate cancer develop among men over the age of 65, but risk starts to increase after age 50. Other risk factors include:

- Having a brother or father with prostate cancer
- Caribbean, African, or African-American ethnicity
- Workplace exposure to toxic substances

dark-skinned individuals absorb less UV rays needed to manufacture vitamin D. Low vitamin D levels are known to increase risk among all men. Some evidence also shows that a low testosterone level increases risk of aggressive types of prostate cancer.

Chronic inflammation is the main causative factor of this cancer. Men with chronic inflammatory diseases of the prostate, such as chronic prostatitis, are at higher risk. The popularity of oral sex will most likely increase risks, as the mouth contains a great number of infectious organisms which can travel along the urethra to the prostate.

Conventional Treatment

In many cases, the only treatment is "watchful waiting," meaning monitoring the condition and if it isn't progressing at a significant rate, doing nothing, because the risks of treatment may be greater than those of the disease. In other cases, surgery, chemotherapy, radiation, hormone therapy, or other treatments may be used.

All prostate cancer treatments destroy the prostate and leave permanent side effects, yet the patient's life may not be seriously impacted by the disease. Consequently, risks of the cancer and risks of treatment always have to be carefully weighed. Recent reviews of radiation treatment of prostate cancer demonstrate not only poor results but also a very high complication rate, the most common being radiation-induced interstitial cystitis, a painful bladder condition, and proctitis, inflammation and pain in the rectum. Both are debilitating. Once the tumor has metastasized, chemotherapy and radiation have little to offer.

👍 My Recommendations

The most important weapon against prostate cancer is the diet. A bad diet can cause chronic inflammation, impair detoxification systems in the liver and in all cells, lower antioxidant defenses, weaken the immune system, and create conditions that increase the likelihood of cancer development, growth, and spread. Over time, a poor diet can also lead to frailty and chronic diseases, which make it more difficult to tolerate treatment if cancer does develop.

The most important dietary elements are described in the "Cancer Basics" section, but there are some additional ones for prostate cancer prevention and to enhance treatment. Diet should consist mostly of cruciferous vegetables, as these inhibit prostate cancer. Other good anticancer plant foods include onions, garlic, greens, spinach, celery, and parsley. Blenderized vegetables are best. Breads and other foods containing gluten should be eaten only in limited amounts and avoided altogether if one is gluten-sensitive or already has a tumor.

For a healthy prostate, it's vital to drink liquids throughout the day to improve lymphatic drainage and circulation in tiny microvessels that deliver blood to tissues. White and green teas are the best beverages because they contain powerful inhibitors of prostate cancer and reduce absorption of harmful heme iron from meat. Glutamate, as found in MSG and other excitotoxin additives, should be avoided because it can stimulate the growth and invasion of prostate and other cancers. For different ways in which it is disguised on food labels, see the chapter "Excitotoxins."

Avoid smoking and the use of nicotine patches, as nicotine lowers immunity and thus increases cancer risk. Also avoid exposure to other toxins, including pesticides, herbicides, industrial chemicals, automobile exhaust fumes, radon gases, and toxic metals such as aluminum, lead, mercury, arsenic, cadmium, and manganese.

Exercise is also important and has been shown to reduce the risk of most cancers. This can include brisk walking, resistance exercises, bike riding, or other moderately vigorous activity. Sedentary lifestyles increase the risk of frailty, chronic inflammation, depression, and poor immune function. Exercise at least for 30 minutes, four to five times a week. Resistance exercise, which should work all the major muscles, is critical but often overlooked. It strengthens muscles, tendons, and ligaments, improves blood flow, improves lymphatic drainage and circulation, boosts our internal antioxidant function, reduces depression, increases energy levels, and improves the immune system.

Stress is a major source of inflammation and damaging free radicals. It can be mental or physical stress—especially if it involves a lack of sleep. Quality sleep is essential for good health and especially immune function. As we get older, we produce less of the sleep-inducing hormone melatonin, which has been shown to reduce cancer risk and can be taken as a supplement. If sleep is problematic, I prefer using the lowest dose of a sublingual melatonin supplement, around 0.5 mg, 30 minutes before bedtime.

Stress can be reduced in multiple ways, including: maintaining close family ties, socializing, having strong religious beliefs, attending your place of worship, listening to beautiful or inspiring music, watching enjoyable movies, or taking a vacation.

A healthy detoxification system strengthens resistance to cancers, as it cleanses the body of toxins, both from the environment and from the byproducts of one's metabolism. When detoxification is impaired, it is most often the result of a poor diet, which can be corrected. Detoxification takes place in the liver and in each cell in the body and can be improved by some supplements, such as quercetin, naringenin, and indole-3-carbinol, described below.

Natural Supplements
▶ Flaxseed Hull Lignans
Lignans are a therapeutic component of flaxseed. Bacteria in the colon convert compounds in the seed into powerful inhibitors

of prostate cancer. I prefer Flax Hull Lignans, made by Progressive Labs.

> ➠ **What to do:** Take one to two level tablespoons of Flax Hull Lignans, once or twice daily. Each dose contains 1.5 g of lignans. The powder can be added to a blenderized vegetable drink or mixed with water, juice, or goat's milk.

▶ DHA

Fish oil contains two key beneficial fats: EPA and DHA, and both reduce inflammation. However, DHA has the more powerful anticancer effects for preventing and reducing growth of the cancer. DHA comes from algae, which is eaten by fish.

> ➠ **What to do:** Take 500 to 700 mg of DHA daily, in a fish oil or algae supplement.

▶ Curcumin

The herbal extract is a powerful inhibitor of prostate cancer. In addition, it enhances the cancer-killing effects of chemotherapy and radiation treatments, while protecting surrounding healthy tissue in the pelvis and rectum. It also inhibits angiogenesis, which is the growth of blood vessels that feed a tumor, and can reverse multidrug resistance. Equally important, it has been shown to reduce the metastasis of prostate cancer to the bones, a very common site of spread.

> ➠ **What to do:** For best absorption, use CurcumaSorb, made by Pure Encapsulations, which contains 250 mg per capsule. For protection, take 250 mg, twice a day with meals. Higher doses have been recommended for treatment of prostate cancer—up to 1,000 mg, three to four times a day with food.

▶ Quercetin

Found in plants, quercetin inhibits the growth and spread of various types of prostate cancer and can reverse multidrug resistance. It is a powerful antioxidant and anti-inflammatory, especially when taken with curcumin, and enhances the effectiveness of treatment while protecting healthy tissue. When combined with green tea, or a green tea extract such as Teavigo (see below), quercetin enhances the killing power of docetaxel, a common chemotherapy drug for prostate cancer.

> ▶ **What to do:** For prevention, take 250 mg, two to three times a day with meals. Treatment requires higher doses, up to 1,000 mg, three times a day with meals. Quercenase, made by Thorne Research, is a well-absorbed form. If you use another brand, where capsules contain a powder, break them open and mix the powder with fish oil to increase absorption.

▶ Teavigo

A standardized extract from green tea, Teavigo contains exceptionally high concentrations of EGCG, the therapeutic ingredient in the tea, and inhibits prostate cancer in a number of ways. It is especially powerful at inhibiting some of the most invasive prostate cancers and can reduce muscle loss that commonly accompanies cancer. The extract is even more effective when combined with quercetin. EGCG also enhances the effectiveness of doxorubicin, a chemotherapy drug used in prostate cancer treatment.

> ▶ **What to do:** For prevention, take one capsule of Teavigo (100 mg) daily with a meal. During treatment, take one capsule, three times a day with meals. Anyone who has documented liver damage or takes medications that damage the liver should not take Teavigo or any other EGCG supplement.

▶ Silymarin

Studies have shown that this extract of the milk thistle plant increases the cancer-killing power of chemotherapy agents, inhibits cancer invasion and spread, and increases self-destruction (apoptosis) of prostate cancer cells. Its ability to enhance liver function, especially detoxification, is of major importance in prostate cancer treatment.

⮞ **What to do:** Silymarin is poorly absorbed as a powder. To improve absorption, mix the contents of capsules with a tablespoon of fish oil or extra virgin olive oil. Or, use Siliphos, made by Thorne Research, which is a well absorbed form. Take 200 mg, twice a day with food.

▶ Indole-3-carbinol (I3C) or DIM

Indole-3-carbinol, or I3C for short, is found in high concentrations in cruciferous vegetables, especially Brussels sprouts and broccoli. DIM (short for diindolylmethane) is another form of the compound. In the human body, either form can be converted to the other. DIM inhibits tumor invasion and enhances chemotherapy against androgen-sensitive and the more aggressive androgen-insensitive prostate cancers. Indole-3-carbinol has been shown to enhance the effectiveness of radiation treatments for prostate cancer.

⮞ **What to do:** Use either indole-3-carbinol or DIM. I suggest taking 100 mg of DIM, three times a day with meals, in DIM-Pro 100, made by Pure Encapsulations, as it has been tested in studies. Or, take 400 mg of indole-3-carbinol, three times a day with meals.

▶ Berberine

This natural plant compound inhibits inflammation, growth of cancer cells, and invasion of prostate cancer into surrounding healthy tissues. In addition, it reduces harmful effects of chemotherapy on surrounding normal tissue, enhances radiation treatment, and reduces risk of metastasis.

⮞ **What to do:** Take 500 mg, three times a day with meals. Berberine-500, made by Thorne Research, is a good quality product. One caution: in people with a history of reactive hypoglycemia, berberine can cause headaches.

▶ Apigenin and Naringenin

Studies have found that apigenin, a flavonoid found in higher concentrations in celery and parsley, is a superior anticancer agent. It suppresses inflammation, inhibits prostate cancer growth, reduces its spread, and inhibits angiogenesis, meaning the growth of blood vessels that support tumors. In addition, apigenin makes cancer cells more sensitive to radiation treatment while protecting surrounding healthy cells. It works even better when combined with naringenin, also in the flavonoid family of nutrients, found in grapefruit and other citrus fruits.

> ➡ **What to do:** For prevention, take 50 to 100 mg of apigenin, two to three times a day. During treatment, take up to 1,000 mg of apigenin, three times a day, with or without food. For prevention or treatment, take 500 mg of naringenin, three times a day with meals.

▶ Luteolin

This is a flavonoid found in higher concentrations in celery, onion leaves, parsley, peppers, broccoli, cabbage, and carrots. Studies have shown it to be a potent cancer inhibitor by interfering with a number of cell-signaling pathways that support cancer cells. It is also a powerful inhibitor of tumor invasion and cancer spread, and sensitizes prostate cancer cells to radiation treatment while protecting surrounding healthy cells. I recommend the Luteolin Complex from Swanson.

> ➡ **What to do:** The most effective dose has not been precisely determined but a reasonable one would be 100 mg, three times a day, and up to 1,000 mg, three times a day. It can be taken with or without food.

▶ Hyperbaric Oxygen Therapy (HBOT)

Hyperbaric oxygen therapy has not been documented in medical literature as a treatment for prostate cancer, but since HBOT inhibits inflammation and enhances killing of many types of cancer cells, one would suspect it would be a useful tool. It is an excellent way to treat two of the most serious complications of radiation treatment of prostate cancer: radiation-induced hemorrhagic cystitis, a painful bladder condition, and proctitis, inflammation of the rectum.

CHAPTER 12

Skin and Hair

Acne

Most common in teenagers, acne can also occur in adults and younger children. Although it is most noticeable on the face, it can also appear on the neck, back, chest, and shoulders. Generally referred to as pimples, acne can manifest as red inflamed cysts on the skin, blackheads, or whiteheads. When acne develops, pores on the surface of the skin become clogged, as a result of too much oil being produced by glands, and dirt and bacteria can then become trapped. Sometimes, acne can develop under the skin as cysts that are hard and painful.

From a conventional medical perspective, the exact cause is unknown. Hormonal changes are believed to play a role during puberty, pregnancy, menstrual cycles, as a result of stress, or in conjunction with taking birth control pills. However, newer research shows that acne is not just a skin problem, but often begins in the intestines, where underlying inflammation is triggered.

Conventional Treatment

For anyone with acne, it is generally recommended to keep skin and hair clean and avoid oily cleansers, creams, and hair care products. Acne medications and prescription creams are designed to kill bacteria and dry out excess oil, and sometimes make skin peel.

Chemical skin peels and photodynamic therapy (PDT) are other possible treatments. In PDT, a light-sensitizing topical lotion or cream is applied to the skin and then a light with a specific wavelength is used to selectively destroy infected tissue.

My Recommendations

In 1911, a gastroenterologist concluded that "toxemia" from an inflamed colon was causing acne. Research since then has supported this premise, showing that bacterial overgrowth and digestive malfunction lead to inflammation in the body that manifests as acne and inflammation in the brain that leads to depression and anxiety, which are more common among people suffering from acne. As one example of the digestive connection, some 40 percent of people with acne have low stomach acid, which leads to overgrowth of harmful bacteria that trigger and perpetuate inflammation.

Another underlying mechanism is leaky gut, whereby harmful bacteria and food particles can leak through the wall of the intestine and directly enter the bloodstream. This causes an antibody reaction that leads to inflammation throughout the body. Problems with constipation are also

---

ACNE TRIGGERS

Any of these can contribute to acne:

- Hormonal changes
- Estrogen or testosterone prescriptions
- Steroid drugs
- Phenytoin, a type of anti-convulsive drug

---

common in people with acne, again linking gut problems with the skin disorder.

Long-term antibiotics have been a mainstay of the medical profession in treating acne, but these have dire side effects. They destroy probiotics, the beneficial bacteria in the digestive system, and suppress our immune defenses against infections. Several recent studies show that correcting deficiencies in probiotics can improve and even cure acne in a high percentage of people. In addition, this helps relieve anxiety and depression, which skin lotions and antibiotics cannot do.

Diet is another important factor, with most studies showing that processed foods, sugar, high-starch carbohydrates, and inflammatory fats greatly increase risk. Milk from cows raised with bovine growth hormone, which is absorbed when we drink their milk, can be another trigger. If you drink milk, organic is a better option.

Natural Supplements
▶ Probiotics and Prebiotics

Probiotics are the friendly bacteria normally found in the colon, and prebiotics are substances that feed these organisms. Both Lactobacillus and Bifidobacterium species of probiotics have been shown to be beneficial for treating and preventing acne. For example, Lactobacillus paracasei has been shown to reduce skin inflammation associated with high levels of a substance in the skin that increases sebum production, which forms pustules. Lactobaccillus rhamnosus has been shown to reduce anxiety and stress, both playing major roles in acne.

Quality is important when choosing probiotic supplements. I recommend Theralac, made by Master Supplements. It contains probiotics and prebiotics, and the live organisms remain viable for six months at room temperature, and up to two years if refrigerated.

Probiotics are also beneficial when applied topically, in soaps and lotions. Several studies have shown that they increase skin levels of ceramides, substances that are naturally present in cell membranes and help to reduce inflammation and harmful bacteria in skin.

➡ **What to do:** Take one capsule of Theralac daily for three months, and then one capsule twice a week. Cleanse with Dr. Ohhira's Probiotic Kampuku Beauty Bar Soap.

▶ **Vitamin A and Zinc**

People with acne have been shown to have very low levels of vitamin A in their skin. As high doses of vitamin A can be toxic, the safest ways to supplement it is by taking mixed carotenoids, several of which are converted into vitamin A in the skin. Zinc is also frequently in short supply.

➡ **What to do:** Take 10,000 to 15,000 IU of mixed carotenoids a day. For severe cases, go up to 25,000 IU a day. Take 30 mg daily of Zinc Picolinate, made by Thorne Research.

▶ **Silver Solutions**

Silver is an excellent antibacterial, antiviral, and antifungal agent for topical treatment of bacterial and viral skin infections. With acne, none of the harmful organisms develop resistance to silver, as they do to antibiotics. I do not recommend taking silver orally.

➡ **What to do:** Apply a silver solution topically to affected areas of skin, per product directions.

▶ **Hyperbaric Oxygen Therapy (HBOT)**

HBOT is known to kill bacteria in infected tissues, especially deep-seated infection such as we see in acne. While I am not aware of it being used to treat acne, it should be of significant benefit.

Athlete's Foot

Caused by a fungus, athlete's foot manifests as red, itchy, burning skin that may crack, become scaly, or develop blisters. Most often, it occurs between the toes, but can also affect the heel and bottom of the foot, fingers, nails, and other parts of the body. It isn't limited to athletes.

Conventional Treatment

Antifungal creams and powders are available without a prescription. Athlete's foot can disappear and then return, without new exposure to the fungus. If it lasts more than a few weeks, leads to swelling or fever, or occurs in someone who has diabetes or a weak immune system, medical treatment may include prescription antifungal medication.

HOW ATHLETE'S FOOT SPREADS

The fungus that causes athlete's food thrives in warm, dark, damp areas such as showers, locker room floors, and areas surrounding swimming pools. Warm, sweaty feet in shoes and socks enable the fungus to grow and survive. It can also be transmitted by sharing footwear. Scratching an infected foot and then touching other parts of the body can spread the fungus to those areas, especially ones that tend to get moist.

My Recommendations

Feet should be kept clean and dry. Socks made of natural fibers and shoes made with real leather are recommended because they provide better ventilation than synthetic materials. Or, open shoes or sandals will provide ventilation, if the climate allows. Natural remedies can help to fight and prevent athlete's foot from the inside as well as topically.

Natural Supplements

▶ Aged Garlic Extract

Garlic is a powerful antifungal agent and, unlike many pharmaceutical agents, can be used for very long periods. Taken internally, it can improve healing and resistance to further athlete's foot outbreaks. Kyolic Aged Garlic Extract, made by Wakunaga, is an odorless garlic extract with consistent high quality and potency.

➡ **What to do:** Take two capsules of Kyolic Aged Garlic Extract 100% Vegetarian Cardiovascular Formula 100, twice a day with meals.

▶ Tea Tree Oil

Tea tree oil has very powerful antifungal properties. It is as effective as many dangerous and costly pharmaceutical medications and can even clear tough, deep-seated infections of toenails and fingernails. Make sure that any product you buy is 100 percent pure tea tree oil.

➡ **What to do:** First, wash the affected area thoroughly with soap and water and dry it well. Put a few drops of tea tree oil on a moist cotton pad and apply it to infected skin, three to four times daily.

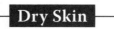

Dry Skin

Most often, dry skin is a minor discomfort and may be a cosmetic concern, but if it becomes lasting or severe, scratching itchy areas can lead to thickening, darkening, cracking, and bacterial infections. Most common in the hands, arms, and lower legs, dry skin is more common among older people because, with age, the skin becomes thinner and pores produce less oils. Changes in hormones, especially a deficiency in thyroid hormone, can also result in dry skin.

Conventional Treatment

The simplest home treatment includes using a moisturizer, avoiding harsh cleansers, and installing a humidifier if the air is dry in your home. Where dryness is severe or skin is swollen or inflamed, prescription creams may be used. Avoid prolonged hot showers. If the condition is persistent, a doctor should check if the dryness is a side effect of medications or if there is an underlying medical condition.

👍 My Recommendations

An inflammatory diet, high in sugar and omega-6 oils such as corn, safflower, sunflower, peanut, and soybean oils, can dry out skin. A diet high in nutrient-dense vegetables, such as cauliflower, Brussels sprouts, broccoli, greens, squash, leeks, and some garlic can protect the skin and help reduce inflammation and dryness. The anti-inflammatory diet in chapter 1 and the vegetable drink in chapter 3 are recommended.

WHAT DRIES OUT SKIN
Although some people are prone to dry skin, especially as they get older, these are common contributors:
• Taking baths or showers for more than 5 to 7 minutes
• Living in a dry climate
• Dry indoor air
• Using harsh cleansers
• Working with harsh chemicals
• Having an occupation that requires frequent hand washing
• Having a skin disease as a child
• Side effects of some drugs
• Underlying medical conditions, such as hypothyroidism

Often, a deficiency in omega-3 oils, those found in fish, is a cause of dry skin. And, a combination of nutrients, such as those in a multivitamin and mineral supplement, all help to make skin healthier.

🐟 Natural Supplements

▶ Fish Oil

Omega-3 fats in fish oil are anti-inflammatory and help to keep skin soft, supple, and lubricated. Choose one with both of the major components found naturally in fish oil, DHA and EPA, but look for a high-quality, pure product with higher levels of DHA. One such product is Super DHA Gems, made by Carlson, which contains 500 mg of DHA and 100 mg of EPA per softgel.

➡ **What to do:** Take two softgels of Carlson's Super DHA Gems a day.

▶ Borage Oil

Borage oil contains another type of beneficial fat, gamma linolenic acid, or GLA for short, which helps to keep skin hydrated
and can relieve itching. It can be taken orally as a supplement
and used topically on dry areas.

➡ **What to do:** Take 1,000 mg daily of a borage oil supplement and topically apply a borage oil lotion or cream, such
as Borage Therapy, made by Shikai, on dry areas of skin.

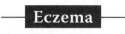

Eczema

An itchy, inflamed, irritating rash, eczema is not a single disease
but a term that describes skin conditions with these symptoms.
The most common one, called atopic eczema (also called atopic
dermatitis), is believed to be a reaction of the immune system,
but its cause is unknown. Eczema is most common in children,
who frequently outgrow it, although it also affects adults. The
condition is often found among people with a family history of
asthma or allergies.

Eczema can occur on almost any area of the skin, but is most
common on the face, scalp, around the ankles, wrists, hands and in-
sides of the elbows. It can prog-
ress into dry, leathery, or inflamed
patches and even blisters. Itching is
a common symptom, and the more
one scratches, the worse the damage to skin.

ECZEMA FLARE-UPS

Eczema can improve and worsen.
For some people, these are triggers
of flare-ups:

- Clothing or bedding made of
  irritating fabrics
- Some soaps, household cleaning
  products, and laundry detergents
- Coming into contact with animal
  dander
- A flare-up of another allergy
- Catching a cold or flu

🔖 Conventional Treatment

Medical treatment aims to reduce the symptoms of eczema.
Over-the-counter and prescription

creams typically contain corticosteroids to reduce inflammation and itching. Antihistamines, ultraviolet light therapy, and immunosuppressant drugs are also used to help quell symptoms. Prescription immunosuppressant creams are also available, but are viewed as a last resort and only for short-term use because they may increase risk for cancer. And, such creams are not approved for children under age 2.

👍 My Recommendations

Whenever possible, identifying and avoiding triggers is a simple way to prevent eczema and help it heal. The most common ones are dust mites, cold, heat, humidity, irritating fabrics, pollen, toxic detergents, excessive stress, food allergies or food intolerance, irritating cosmetic products, pet dander, hot tubs, smoking, and exposure to secondhand smoke.

An anti-inflammatory diet, described in chapter 1, is a mainstay for healthy skin. It's high in vegetables, low in red meat, sugar, and starch, with ample healthy fats and pure water, along with regular exercise. It's also important to avoid herbicides and pesticides in food, beverages, and around the house and garden. In addition, probiotics can quell inflammation and immune reactions that stem from digestive issues. See the "Acne" section for how this works and what to do.

One of the key elements in treating the condition is to suppress mast cell release of histamine and other inflammatory substances, which are major culprits in the severe itching seen with eczema. A number of natural supplements can help to accomplish this.

🐇 Natural Supplements
▶ Green Tea Extract

These teas contain a group of flavonoid compounds that collectively are called catechins. One of the most beneficial is called EGCG, short for epigallocatechin gallate. EGCG is a powerful inhibitor of histamine and reduces itching and redness. I recommend a product called Teavigo, made by Pure Encapsulations. One capsule contains 141 mg.

➠ **What to do:** Take one 141 mg capsule of Teavigo, two to three times a day with meals. On very rare instances, liver damage has been reported in some individuals who take this product. It is not clear why and it is usually reversible once the product is discontinued. As an alternative, drink a cup of white tea, three times a day.

▶ Baicalin

An extract from the skullcap plant, baicalin is a powerful inhibitor of mast cell release of histamine and other inflammatory substances. I recommend using a powdered version called simply Baicalin, made by LiftMode.

➠ **What to do:** Mix ¼ teaspoon of baicalin powder with a tablespoon of extra virgin olive oil and take this mixture three times a day, with meals.

▶ Gamma Linolenic Acid (Borage Oil)

Abbreviated GLA, this is the key beneficial ingredient in borage oil. It has been shown to reduce skin itching and increase moisture levels of skin.

➠ **What to do:** Take 500 mg of GLA, twice a day with meals.

▶ Coconut Oil

Coconut oil has been promoted as a useful agent in treating eczema. It contains an oil called MCT, short for medium chain triglyceride, which is probably the effective component. This oil can be used for cooking and can be taken as a supplement.

➠ **What to do:** Take one tablespoon, three times daily, after meals. If you don't like the taste of coconut, I suggest using refined coconut oil, which has no coconut taste or smell.

▶ Luteolin

A powerful inhibitor of mast cell activation, luteolin reduces itching and skin inflammation. I recommend a product called Luteolin Complex, made by Swanson Health Products.

➡ **What to do:** Take 100 mg, three times a day with meals.

▶ Magnesium

Magnesium is a powerful anti-inflammatory mineral that can be used topically. Add Epsom salt, which is magnesium sulfate, or a magnesium oil to a bath, and see how you feel. Some people get relief while others are irritated by baths. Or, rub magnesium oil or gel onto affected areas of skin.

➡ **What to do:** Add two cups of Epsom salt to a tub of water and have a relaxing soak.

▶ Colostrum

The watery fluid that is secreted by the breast just before milk is released, colostrum contains a number of health-promoting compounds which, with regular use of the supplement, can improve eczema skin lesions by reducing allergic or otherwise excessive immune reactions. I recommend using one of these products: Colostrum LD, made by Sovereign Laboratories, in capsules or as a powder, or an oral spray from the same manufacturer, called IRM (Immune Response Modulator)

➡ **What to do:** Depending upon your personal preference, take capsules or powder, or use the spray, according to the manufacturer's directions.

▶ Hyperbaric Oxygen Therapy (HBOT)

Eczema is a chronic inflammatory skin disease, and since HBOT is known to reduce inflammation, one would expect it to be of benefit. Other inflammatory skin diseases have been shown to improve with HBOT treatments.

Hair Loss

In the United States, an estimated 40 million men and 20 million women experience hair loss. The most common form is androgenic alopecia, or pattern baldness, with different patterns in men and women.

Among men, it begins with a receding hairline and thinning on the crown, and can progress until there is only a ring of hair around the back and sides of the head, and then no hair at all. Women don't usually experience a receding hairline. Instead, there is usually thinning of hair in the front and on the crown of the head.

In conventional medicine, heredity is believed to be a major risk factor, and hormones and age contribute, but the actual cause is unknown. Some medical conditions, such as thyroid disorders, and medications can contribute to this common type of hair loss.

There are several other, less common forms of hair loss. Hair grows in cycles, with each one growing for about two years and then resting for about two months. Normally, about 80 to 90 percent of our hair follicles are in the growth phase producing new hair, but when they get stuck in the no-growth phase, it leads to hair loss. The fancy medical term for this is "telogen effluvium." It appears to be related to stress, exposure to environmental toxins, and poor nutrition.

Patchy loss of hair, technically called alopecia areata, may stem from an immune reaction. It can resolve by itself but sometimes progresses to loss of all body hair, which is called alopecia totalis. Certain vaccinations are known to be associated with this condition, especially the hepatitis B vaccine.

A related but rarer condition is scarring alopecia, technically called cicatricial alopecia, which involves scarring of sections of the scalp with loss of hair. It is more common among women. The scarring is usually in the front of the scalp and can be quite severe and disfiguring. The cause is not known, but appears to be an intense immune reaction involving the hair follicle. It can be painful, with an intense burning and redness of the scalp.

In all forms of hair loss, the common denominator appears to be inflammation around the hair follicle, and immune reactions may also play a part. In body builders and sports enthusiasts who use high-dose testosterone products, high concentrations of the hormone are known to induce inflammation, which can lead to hair loss.

Conventional Treatment

Medically recognized treatments for pattern baldness include hair transplants and these:

Topical foams and lotions: Rogaine and minoxidil, the generic form, are available without a prescription, for men and women. These need to be applied to the scalp twice daily, and work only as long as the treatment is continued. Itching or irritation are common side effects, but breathing problems or growth of unwanted facial hair are among other, less frequent adverse reactions.

HAIR LOSS FACTS
Noticeable hair loss affects:
Men
By age 35: 40%
By age 50: 50%
By age 60: 65%
By age 80: 70%
By age 85: 80%
Women
By age 40: 40%
By age 60: 50%
By age 80: 55%

Prescription medications: Proscar, Propecia, and the generic form, finasteride, are usually prescribed only for men. They were originally developed to treat an enlarged prostate, but hair growth was also observed among some men in clinical trials. To maintain any new hair growth, the drugs need to be taken for life. Sexual problems, depression, and suicidal thoughts can be side effects, even months after the drugs are discontinued.

For scarring alopecia, steroid injections into the scalp are the only conventional treatment. It may slow the progress of the condition in some women, but for many it has little effectiveness and can have complications.

👍 My Recommendations

Because there are various causes of hair loss, it is impossible to pinpoint a single agent that can prevent it. Overall good nutrition, which is described in the chapter "The Anti-Aging Prescription," is recommended, as it reduces overall chronic inflammation. Avoiding excitotoxins, as described in the "Excitotoxins" chapter, helps to prevent and reduce autoimmune reactions. Blenderizing vegetables, as described in the "Drink Your Veggies" chapter, is a simple way to get concentrated plant nutrients that reduce the odds of both inflammation and auto-immune reactions.

In male and female pattern baldness, too much testosterone is converted to a form called dihydrotestosterone, or DHT for short, in the hair follicle. An enzyme called 5 alpha-reductase enables this conversion to take place. Drugs such as Proscar, Propecia, and the generic form, finasteride, inhibit this enzyme but can also cause side effects and may not be effective, as the hair loss may be due to factors other than DHT. Some herbs and nutrients can inhibit the same enzyme or block binding of DHT to hair follicles. Low thyroid can also underlie hair loss, especially in women, and should be checked for by a health professional.

Scarring alopecia affects mostly women. It may stem from a combination of genetics, use of toxic hair products, other exposure to environmental toxins, and an autoimmune mechanism, meaning the immune system attacks some hair follicles. Chemicals in hair products, including dyes, should be avoided by using non-toxic products. Heat, from hair dryers and styling tools, should also be avoided, as it can worsen inflammation and damage to hair follicles.

Studies of scarring alopecia have found a common defect in a special anti-inflammatory cell-signaling system called PPAR-γ (peroxisome proliferator-activated receptor-gamma) within the stem cells of hair follicles. Some natural supplements, such as luteolin, quercetin, baicalein, and DHA, can restore the activity of this anti-inflammatory system.

Natural Supplements

▶ Pattern Baldness

Natural substances that can inhibit DHT or block it from binding to hair follicles include pygeum, saw palmetto, bladderwrack, beta-sitosterol, and gamma linolenic acid (GLA), a beneficial fat found in some plant oils, such as borage oil and evening primrose oil. Some formulas contain a combination of some of these, along with other nutrients. Hairomega DHT, made by Bioprosper, is one such product. It includes saw palmetto, pygeum, and beta-sitosterol but also contains some mushroom extracts, which can worsen autoimmune-related hair loss. Hairomega 3-in-1, also made by Bioprosper, does not contain mushroom extracts and contains saw palmetto and beta-sitosterol. All these products are for men and women. Vitamin D3 may also help.

Another approach is to use topical formulas with some of these same ingredients. Revivogen MD Scalp Therapy, made by Revivogen, is a topical scalp serum with saw palmetto, GLA, and other beneficial ingredients.

⮞ **What to do:** Take separate supplements of saw palmetto, pygeum, beta-sitosterol, and GLA, per product directions, or take a formula such as one of the Hairomega products. Use the Revivogen scalp serum by itself or along with dietary supplements. For vitamin D3, it's best to get blood levels tested and take the amount needed to achieve and maintain blood levels between 35 and 100 ng/ml. Topical vitamin D3 products can also be used.

▶ Autoimmune Hair Loss

Several natural substances can increase PPAR-γ, the body's anti-inflammatory system that is defective in cases of scarring alopecia or other autoimmune-related hair loss. These include luteolin, quercetin, baicalein, and DHA. In addition, in all such cases, vitamin D3 is a powerful immune modulator—meaning that it helps prevent autoimmune reactions. It is most effective when used topically, but oral vitamin D3 is also helpful.

➡ **What to do:** Use a topical vitamin D3 product. Get blood levels of vitamin D3 tested and take enough to achieve and maintain blood levels between 35 and 100 ng/ml. These are doses for the other nutrients: 50 mg of luteolin, three times a day with meals; 500 mg of quercetin, in a well-absorbed product called Quercenase, made by Thorne Research, three times a day with meals; 1,000 mg daily of DHA, from fish oil or algae. For baicalein, take a product called Baicalin, made by LiftMode, ¼ teaspoon of the powder mixed with a tablespoon of extra virgin olive oil, three times a day with meals.

▶ Hyperbaric Oxygen Therapy (HBOT)

There are no studies showing that this treatment cures hair loss, but I have heard of some cases where HBOT treatment centers reported that hair growth was stimulated. One of the causes of hair loss, especially in women, is an inflammatory autoimmune disorder called cicatricial alopecia, or scarring alopecia, which not only causes hair loss but also varying degrees of scarring of the scalp. HBOT, as an inflammatory treatment, should be of benefit for this condition.

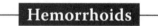

Hemorrhoids

Hemorrhoids are swollen veins in the anal canal or near its opening. They afflict about half of men and women after the age of 50, may or may not be painful, and bleed during bowel movements. Those that occur outside the anus may make it difficult to clean the area and can develop into a painful blood clot.

Hemorrhoids often go away without treatment but when they form clots, these can kill nearby tissue, which may need to be removed by a doctor. Hemorrhoids can also cause uncomfortable itching and pain while sitting. Straining while having a bowel movement is believed to be a major trigger.

> **HEMORRHOID SYMPTOMS**
>
> Signs include:
> - Bleeding from the rectum, visible on stool, in the toilet bowl, or on toilet paper
> - Painful bowel movements
> - Itching
> - Pain or discomfort while sitting
> - Bumps just inside or near the rectum

Conventional Treatment

Over-the-counter creams can dull pain and reduce swelling, and products designed to soften stools can decrease irritation and help hemorrhoids heal. At the doctor, the first step of diagnosis is a rectal exam. Scopes can also be used to look inside the rectum, and biopsies can be done to check for more serious conditions, such as cancerous polyps.

Hemorrhoids can be surgically removed with a scalpel, or a staple or rubber band may be used to block blood flow to the swollen tissue, causing it to shrink. After any of these treatments, doctors usually recommend drinking lots of fluids, eating only soft foods, and using a stool softener, to avoid irritating bowel movements while the area is healing.

My Recommendations

Hemorrhoids are rectal veins that have weak walls, which lead to engorgement of the veins. Natural products that strengthen the walls of these veins will, in most cases, cure the condition, but it is also important to avoid constipation, which is a common cause of hemorrhoids.

A diet high in vegetable fiber will not only relieve constipation, but will also reduce your risk of colon and rectal cancer. The drink in chapter 3 makes it easy to get those extra vegetables and fiber. Most important is hydration, which is a special problem in the elderly. Dehydration hardens the stool and reduces mucous production by the rectum, which is necessary for normal bowel movements.

Natural Supplements

▶ Hesperidin and Diosmin

Hesperidin is found in relatively high concentrations in oranges, and diosmin is another form of the same plant compound. Each works in a slightly different, complementary way, and both have been shown to be very effective in strengthening veins.

➡ **What to do:** Take 1,000 mg of hesperidin, three times daily, until the hemorrhoids subside, then take a maintenance dose of 500 mg twice a day. It can be taken without food. At the same time, take 500 to 600 mg of diosmin daily. Look for Diosmin 95 as an ingredient on product labels.

▶ Vitamin C

A deficiency of vitamin C is a common cause of weak veins, as the vitamin is essential for building tissue in the supporting walls of veins. High doses of vitamin C can reduce the incidence of hemorrhoid attacks and, in many cases, eliminate them altogether. To avoid stomach upset, it's best to take a buffered form of vitamin C, listed on ingredient labels as calcium ascorbate or magnesium ascorbate. Or, take a highly absorbable product called Lypo-Spheric Vitamin C, made by LivOn Labs, which comes in single-serve gel packets that are mixed with water or juice. Each packet contains 1,000 mg of vitamin C.

➡ **What to do:** Take 1,000 mg, three times daily, of a buffered form of vitamin C. Or, take one packet of Lypo-Spheric Vitamin C, twice daily. With both products, always take them between meals, as taking high doses of vitamin C with food can increase iron absorption to unhealthy levels.

Psoriasis

A chronic skin condition that may temporarily get better and then worse, psoriasis manifests as patches of thickened or raised red skin with some silvery-white areas, which are dead skin cells. Its cause is unknown and there is no cure, but it is believed to be an autoimmune disease, where a defective immune system mistakenly attacks healthy skin cells and makes them grow too quickly.

Psoriasis can occur on any part of the body but is more common on the knees, elbows, face, back, neck, scalp, feet, and palms of the hands. It is not possible to catch psoriasis from another person, but some people may have a genetic predisposition for the disease. In some cases, psoriasis may lead to psoriatic arthritis.

> **COMMON PSORIASIS TRIGGERS**
>
> Eruptions of psoriasis may be triggered by a number of things and can vary among individuals. These are some possible ones:
> - Any type of bacterial or viral infection
> - Cuts
> - Burns
> - Insect bites
> - Some prescription drugs
> - Sunburn
> - Lack of exposure to sunlight
> - Drinking too much alcohol
> - Treatments of conditions that weaken the immune system, such as chemotherapy
> - Other disorders of the immune system
> - A dry environment

Conventional Treatment

On the skin surface, various creams, lotions, or ointments can help to soothe skin, moisturize it, and remove scaly patches, and anti-dandruff shampoo can help with psoriatic patches on the scalp. Some of these are available over-the-counter, and others, which are stronger require a prescription.

Internally, doctors may prescribe medications that suppress the immune system. Newer drugs, called biologics, are designed to block a specific type of immune reaction that leads to fast growth of the skin cells that make up the telltale patches of psoriasis. If there is an underlying infection, an antibiotic or antiviral drug may be prescribed. These drugs have a high complication rate and some can increase the risk of developing cancer.

👍 My Recommendations

Psoriasis indicates chronic inflammation, which also underlies heart disease, stroke, diabetes, and other chronic ills, so it is important to reduce the underlying inflammation. Diet is very important and should consist of at least five to ten servings of vegetables with a small amount of fruits (see chapter 3 for how to easily increase your intake) and few inflammatory foods, as in the diet in chapter 1. The worst offenders are sugar, high-starch carbohydrates, inflammatory omega-6 oils, such as corn, safflower, sunflower, peanut, and soybean oils, aspartame in zero-calorie artificial sweeteners, and processed foods containing glutamate additives, such as MSG (see chapter 2).

Other inflammatory substances include fluoride, pesticides in food and around the garden, and toxic chemicals in household products. All these should be avoided.

🐾 Natural Supplements

▶ **Niacinamide**

This form of niacin does not cause any uncomfortable type of flushing reaction. Studies have shown that it dramatically reduces inflammation and improves energy production by all cells. Niacinamide combats psoriasis through multiple mechanisms which reduce inflammation in the skin and lower histamine levels.

➡ **What to do:** Take one 500-mg capsule, two to three times a day with meals, depending on the severity of the condition. For very severe cases, the dose may need to be as high as 2,000 mg, three times a day.

▶ **Coleus Forskohlii**

An extract from the root of a plant that is native to southern Asia, coleus forskohlii contains a plant chemical called forskolin. The extract reduces overgrowth of skin cells, a mechanism that leads to skin lesions in psoriasis.

➡ **What to do:** Take one to two 50-mg capsules, three times a day on an empty stomach.

▶ **Apigenin**

A member of the flavonoid category of nutrients, apigenin is found in a number of edible plants, such as parsley, thyme, peppermint, olives, and chamomile. Studies have shown that apigenin can block autoimmune reactions, reduce inflammation, and improve conditions triggered by these mechanisms, such as psoriasis, rheumatoid arthritis, and Crohn's disease.

➡ **What to do:** Take two 50-mg capsules, three times a day with meals.

▶ **Teavigo**

Teavigo is a concentrated extract of a substance found in green and white tea, EGCG. It has been shown to inhibit autoimmune reactions and reduce inflammation, and it can be taken in capsules or used topically.

➡ **What to do:** Take 100 mg, twice a day, with or without meals. In addition, you can break open a capsule and mix the contents with a lotion or cream and apply it to affected areas of skin.

▶ **GLA (Gamma-Linolenic Acid)**

GLA, short for gamma-linolenic acid, is a naturally occurring oil found in certain seeds, such as evening primrose and borage. Studies have shown that taking GLA daily can improve skin hydration, reduce itching, and improve the skin's barrier protection.

➡ **What to do:** Take 500 mg, twice a day with meals.

▶ **Hesperidin and Hesperidin Plus Vitamin C**

One study found significant benefits supplementing with hesperidin, especially when combined with vitamin C.

➡ **What to do:** Take hesperidin 500 mg three times a day with meals. Buffered vitamin C in a dose of 1,000 mg can be taken three times a day between meals.

▶ **Hyperbaric Oxygen Therapy (HBOT)**

I am not aware of any studies that have tested HBOT as a treatment for psoriasis. However, since psoriasis is an inflammatory skin disorder, and HBOT is known to reduce inflammation, it should produce benefits.

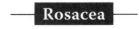

Rosacea

Most often visible as chronic or recurring redness in the cheeks and nose, symptoms can also include red, hot, tender bumps, which sometimes contain pus, and a red nose that looks enlarged and bulbous, especially among men. When rosacea develops, small blood vessels under the skin have become swollen and may have a spider-like appearance, which is technically called telangiectasia.

Rosacea can also affect the eyes, sometimes before it becomes evident in the skin. About half of those who suffer from rosacea have irritated, reddish eyelids, and experience dry eyes. Sometimes, it only affects the eyes.

Conventional Treatment

There is no cure for rosacea. While not life-threatening nor a precursor to a more serious condition, rosacea can be debilitating because of its appearance. Treatment options may include antibiotic creams or lotions that reduce inflammation, but these are only advised for short-term use and may cause problematic side effects.

If there are bumps that look like acne, then acne drugs may be prescribed, but these also have side effects, and can cause birth defects if taken during pregnancy. Cosmetically, laser and light treatments, and some peels, can reduce the appearance of rosacea, although the effects may be temporary.

👍 My Recommendations

The cause of rosacea is not fully understood, but in many cases there is an overgrowth of a microscopic mite in the skin and an abnormal immune reaction to it. Inflammation and immune abnormalities are common denominators. Remedies that reduce skin inflammation with the use of targeted topical treatments can help to reduce symptoms.

> **WHO IS AT RISK?**
>
> Women are more likely than men to suffer from rosacea, especially those who are fair skinned, who blush easily, and are between the ages of 30 and 60. However, men may experience more severe symptoms, and are more likely to develop an enlarged, red nose, sometimes referred to as "the W. C. Fields nose."

🌿 Natural Supplements

▶ Skin Treatments

Several products have been developed, and one with the best reviews is called Redness Relief Kit, made by Zenmed. It is a combination of three products: a gentle cleanser, a serum, and a spray to deliver nutrients to the skin. Although these products are effective, they are fairly expensive.

Anyone on a budget can make skin creams at home by breaking open capsules of key ingredients and mixing their contents with a cream base. The base I have had the most success with is called Derma e Vitamin E Intensive Therapy Body Lotion, made by Derma e. These are the ingredients that, in my experience, would be the most effective:

Teavigo: This is a concentrated version of EGCG, a component of green and white tea that has been shown in a number of studies to reduce skin inflammation, redness, and development of spider veins.

Silymarin: It has been shown to be one of the more effective compounds to treat skin conditions, reduce spider veins, and prevent skin cancer. Silymarin has a slight brown color, which blends well with skin.

MSM: Some studies have shown that a combination of MSM and silymarin in a cream significantly reduce redness and pustule formation.

➡ **What to do:** Use 4 ounces of the Derma e cream as a base and mix it well with the contents of two capsules of Teavigo. For a more effective formula, add contents of two 200-mg capsules of silymarin (a total of 400 mg), and contents of a capsule of MSM. You can use this mixture on all areas of the face.

Shingles

A very painful skin rash that has a blister-like appearance, shingles comes from the same virus that causes chickenpox: the varicella-zoster virus. Anyone who has had chickenpox has the possibility of having the virus lying dormant in nerve cells. When the virus is activated, shingles is the result, and it can cause nerve damage, disfiguring skin lesions, and lasting pain, even after the rash disappears. Shingles may affect one or several nerves. Generalized shingles can be a very serious infection and can result in death. Involvement of the nerves of the face can cause disfiguring scarring or, in rare cases, blindness in the affected eye.

In almost all cases, the virus is triggered into activity by a defect in the immune system. In rare cases, a physical injury or even spinal surgery can activate the virus, but even then, there is some immune suppression. Drugs that suppress immunity, such as steroids, tissue-rejection drugs, and nicotine, are common causes for the development of shingles. When the shingles lesions are active, children who come in contact with the affected person can contract typical chickenpox.

🕭 Conventional Treatment

Medications can help to end a shingles attack, but they don't eliminate the virus. Antihistamines may reduce itching when taken in pill form or used as a lotion on affected areas. Antiviral drugs or corticosteroids may be prescribed to subdue symptoms. And Zostrix, an over-the-counter cream with capsaicin, an extract of pepper, may help to relieve pain.

> **SHINGLES SYMPTOMS**
>
> The virus that causes shingles affects the nervous system. In addition to a painful, burning, and/or itchy rash, symptoms may include:
>
> - Feeling generally unwell
> - Swollen glands
> - Joint pain
> - Fever
> - Chills
> - Weak facial muscles and sight, taste, or hearing problems, if the outbreak affects the face

I am frequently asked about the shingles vaccine, especially by older individuals. I do not recommend the vaccine mainly because the natural supplements below, along with a healthy diet, can prevent shingles. Interestingly, a recent dramatic increase in shingles cases, even among the young, has been attributed to the widespread use of the chickenpox vaccine in children. In the vast majority of cases, chickenpox is a very benign childhood disease and natural infection with the chickenpox virus offers lifelong immunity, unlike the vaccine, which lasts no more than five years.

👍 My Recommendations

Diet is very important in preventing shingles. Inflammatory omega-6 fats, such as corn, soybean, peanut, safflower, and sunflower oils, suppress immunity and can increase one's risk of developing shingles or prolong the suffering. A high-sugar diet also suppresses immunity. Chapter 1 outlines what to eat.

Glutamate and aspartame food additives (see chapter 2) should be avoided as well, as they can worsen neurological damage.

Most vegetables, especially cruciferous ones, keep the immune systems strong and help prevent shingles (see chapter 3 for how to easily increase your intake). Foods high in glutamate, such as mushrooms, red meats, tomato sauces and pureed tomatoes, and cheeses, should be avoided, especially if you already have shingles, as glutamate dramatically worsens the pain and inflammation.

Natural Supplements to Prevent Shingles

▶ Astaxanthin

This is one of the carotenoids found in many fruits and vegetables and in certain types of algae. Salmon eat algae that contains astaxanthin and the nutrient gives them their pink color, as well as stamina and protection. It has been shown to repair most cases of age-related immune suppression that makes people susceptible to shingles.

> ➡ **What to do:** Astaxanthin supplements most often contain 4 mg per softgel capsule. Take one capsule, twice a day with meals.

▶ Beta Glucan

Technically called beta-1,3/1,6-glucan, this is an extract from the cell walls of baker's yeast. Beta glucan stimulates what is called cellular immunity, the arm of the immune system most often impaired in age-related immune suppression. It is also the most powerful in killing viruses and keeping them in a dormant state.

> ➡ **What to do:** Once a week, take 250 mg, on an empty stomach with water.

▶ Olive Leaf Extract

In addition to boosting immune defenses, olive leaf extract helps white blood cells to eliminate bacteria and viruses. It also reduces cholesterol, lowers elevated blood pressure, and protects the brain.

➡ **What to do:** Capsules contain different amounts, depending on the brand. Take 500 mg, once a day with a meal.

Natural Supplements to Treat Shingles

The damage and intense pain associated with this virus is due to two main events: inflammation and a release of high levels of glutamate by the body's cells. Glutamate is a neurotransmitter and, when overactivated, causes excitotoxicity, which leads to significant problems described in more detail in chapter 2. The aim of natural treatment is to reduce the inflammation and to make the virus go back into its dormant stage—that is, put the virus to sleep. Healing of the nerves is also promoted by a number of natural products.

▶ Vitamin B12

Vitamin B12, in the methylcobalamin form (which will be listed on labels), not only stimulates nerve repair but also reduces one of the major reasons for the pain—excitotoxicity. It requires a high dose to treat the pain, at least 10,000 mcg a day. Methylcobalamin is best absorbed as a liquid or in a sublingual form: a dissolvable tablet placed under the tongue.

➡ **What to do:** Take 10,000 mcg of a sublingual form, such as methylcobalamin, once a day.

▶ B-Complex

The B vitamins play an important role in nerve health. The best B-complex product will contain all the major B vitamins, such as thiamine, riboflavin, pyridoxine, niacinamide, biotin, and pantothenic acid, in high doses and in their most absorbable form. The product I use is B-Complex Plus, made by Pure Encapsulations.

➡ **What to do:** Take one capsule of B-Complex Plus, twice a day with meals.

▶ Niacinamide

The most usable form of niacin, niacinamide has been shown to powerfully reduce inflammation by lowering the level of many major pro-inflammatory chemicals in our bodies. It also stimulates cellular energy production. The anti-inflammatory effect is dose-related: the higher the dose, the greater the beneficial effect. Unlike niacin, niacinamide is not toxic to the liver in high doses.

➡ **What to do:** When in severe pain from shingles, take 1,000 to 2,000 mg of niacinamide, three times a day with meals.

▶ Hesperidin

A nutrient in the flavonoid category, hesperidin is found in high concentrations in oranges. It reduces inflammation and turns off the powerful inflammatory cells that are responsible for the pain of shingles. It has also been shown to have tranquilizing effects.

➡ **What to do:** Take 500 mg, three times a day, with or without food.

▶ Curcumin and Quercetin

Also in the flavonoid category of plant nutrients, curcumin and quercetin work together, not only to reduce inflammation but also to protect the spinal cord, which can be affected by shingles. They also promote healing of the skin and the involved nerves.

➡ **What to do:** For best absorption, mix the contents of one 250-mg capsule of quercetin and one 250-mg capsule of curcumin with a tablespoon of either extra virgin olive oil or coconut oil. This mixture can be taken three times a day with meals. Or, take special forms of these that are designed to be well absorbed: CurcumaSorb, made by Pure Encapsulations, and Quercenase, made by Thorne Research. One capsule of each contains 250 mg.

▶ **Teavigo**

This extract from green tea, containing concentrated EGCG, has been shown to prevent shingles viruses from reproducing, thus helping to control the infection and driving the virus back into its dormant state. It is also a powerful anti-inflammatory and antioxidant. In very rare instances, EGCG has been linked to liver injury, which reverses when the product is stopped.

➡ **What to do:** Take one 100-mg capsule, twice a day with meals.

▶ **St. John's Wort**

This herbal product has been shown to reduce nerve pain associated with shingles by reducing excitotoxicity, reducing inflammation, and suppressing viral replication. Liquid forms can be applied to the affected skin several times a day. Oral St. John's Wort should not be combined with medications as it can interfere with their metabolism. The product comes either as a powder in a capsule or as a liquid (tincture). Hypericum is the active compound in the herb. Pure Encapsulation makes a purified hypericum product in a 600 mg per capsule dose.

➡ **What to do:** If using the liquid, one can add 5 to 20 drops in water or juice three times a day. The oral dose is one 600 mg capsule two to three times a day with meals.

▶ **Acetyl-L-carnitine**

This natural product has been shown to significantly reduce nerve pain. The full effect takes weeks to maximize. It also has a number of other advantages, such as promoting memory, stimulating brain plasticity, and healing and inhibiting excitotoxicity. It also stimulates a special receptor in the spinal cord that reduces pain.

➡ **What To do:** The usual dose of 500 mg to 1,000 mg taken three times a day on an empty stomach.

▶ Hyperbaric Oxygen Therapy (HBOT)

Studies have shown that the chickenpox virus, which is responsible for shingles, is killed in the high-oxygen atmosphere of HBOT. In addition, HBOT improves the immune reaction against the virus and reduces inflammation, skin blisters, and pain that accompany shingles outbreaks.

CHAPTER 13

Respiratory

- » Allergies
- » Asthma
- » Bronchitis
- » Chronic Obstructive
  Pulmonary Disease (COPD)
- » Colds and Flu
- » Sleep Apnea

Allergies

Allergies are a reaction of the immune system to common substances we all encounter in everyday life, such as certain foods, dust, pet dander, or pollen. Although these are generally harmless, in some people the immune system treats such allergens as harmful invaders and launches an inflammatory defense mechanism that produces uncomfortable symptoms. Common ones include hay fever, wheezing, or coughing; red, itchy, and watery eyes, known as conjunctivitis; patches of itchy, dry skin; or hives.

Food allergies that affect the digestive system can trigger nausea, diarrhea, vomiting, or digestive discomfort. They can also affect how the brain operates, often leading to such problems as difficulty concentrating, mental fog, and even depression and anxiety.

COMMON ALLERGENS

Substances that trigger allergic reactions vary among individuals, but these are some common ones:

- Soy
- Cow's milk
- Shellfish
- Fish
- Tree nuts
- Peanuts and other legumes, such as lentils and other beans
- Wheat
- Dairy
- Eggs
- Pollen
- Pet dander
- Dust mites
- Mold
- Latex
- Penicillin
- Antibiotics containing penicillin
- Bee or wasp stings
- Ants and ticks

Allergies can be life-threatening when they manifest as anaphylactic shock, usually in reaction to a food, medication, or the venom in bee stings. In such situations, blood vessels can dilate to such a degree that a severe drop in blood pressure leads to fainting or shock. Swelling of the tongue or throat and blocked breathing passages can be deadly without treatment.

Food intolerance or sensitivity, to gluten, for example, is a different, delayed reaction of the immune system, which can manifest in a variety of ways that add up to discomfort, fatigue, or a general feeling of being unwell. Because manifestations may not occur immediately and symptoms can vary, such intolerances can be difficult to diagnose. However, they are not immediately life-threatening. While in some cases exposure to even a very small amount of the substance can cause problems, in most instances symptoms depend on the frequency and amount of the offending food that is eaten. Ironically, people may crave the very foods that are causing problems.

Conventional Treatment

An immediate allergic reaction triggers overproduction of the IgE antibody. When an allergen is suspected, skin and/or blood tests may be done to diagnose the allergy. Treatment varies, depending upon the diagnosis.

In some cases, such as contact with latex, avoiding the allergen may be the most practical solution. In others, medications, such as eye drops or nasal sprays for airborne allergens, may be prescribed or over-the-counter forms may be recommended. In some situations, immunotherapy may be done during a period of several years, with injections of purified allergen extracts. Or, other medications may be prescribed. In the case of potentially life-threatening allergies, doctors usually give patients a device for injecting epinephrine in an emergency, such as an EpiPen, to have on hand in daily life.

Until fairly recently, physicians typically ignored more subtle food allergies, often referred to as food sensitivities or intolerances (to gluten, for example), which did not produce an immediate and severe reaction, such as hives or anaphylactic shock. And still, more common yet subtle and delayed symptoms, such as mental fog or extreme fatigue, are often misdiagnosed as mental health problems.

👍 My Recommendations

The most important thing is to avoid offending allergens. This is easier to do with foods or food additives than with airborne allergens, but even with those, high-quality home air filters can make life much more pleasant.

Additives with glutamate, such as MSG (see chapter 2), and foods naturally high in glutamate, such as mushrooms, tomato paste, tomato sauces, red meats, and cheeses, can activate and worsen immune-system reactions and should be avoided. Offending ingredients are often found in most processed foods, so either avoid processed foods altogether or check food labels very carefully. In contrast, nutrient-dense vegetables protect against and reduce allergic reactions because they contain powerful anti-inflammatory substances, including magnesium, which reduce glutamate-induced immune reactions. Magnesium even reduces anaphylactic reactions.

It's also important to vary foods in one's diet, as eating the same every day can increase the risk of eventually developing a sensitivity to those foods. Drinking a cup of strong white tea can reduce allergy symptoms.

Natural Supplements
▶ Magnesium Malate and Citrate
These are two forms of well-absorbed magnesium. For ongoing protection against allergic reactions, I prefer a slow-release magnesium malate called Magnesium w/SRT, made by Jigsaw Health, but to calm an allergy flare-up, a single, immediate-release dose works better.

➡ **What to do:** Ongoing, take two slow-release tablets of Magnesium w/SRT, twice a day with food. To calm acute reactions, use a magnesium citrate or malate product in capsules, which is not slow-release. Empty the contents of four capsules into 6 ounces of water, stir well, and drink.

▶ Vitamin C
High-dose vitamin C powerfully inhibits histamine release from mast cells, the main immune-system cells that cause allergic reactions, and reduces the inflammatory reactions of allergies. It can be a great help for sinus-related and other symptoms. For best absorption, use Lypo-Spheric Vitamin C, made by LivOn Labs, which contains 1,000 mg of vitamin C in one single-serve packet of a gel which gets mixed with water or juice. It works especially well when combined with quercetin (see below). Always take vitamin C without food, as it increases iron absorption, which can lead to iron overload.

➡ **What to do:** Take one packet of Lypo-Spheric Vitamin C, three times a day without food. For more severe allergies, take two packets (2,000 mg of vitamin C), three times a day on an empty stomach.

▶ Quercetin

Quercetin is one of the most common flavonoids, a very beneficial category of nutrients found in edible plants. Multiple studies have demonstrated that it has powerful anti-allergy effects. Use a well-absorbed form called Quercenase, made by Thorne Research.

> ➡ **What to do:** Take one capsule of Quercenase, three times a day with meals. For more severe allergic attacks, increase each dose to two capsules.

▶ Luteolin

This is a flavonoid found in high concentrations in celery and artichoke. Multiple studies have shown that it powerfully inhibits the release of histamine and other allergy-inducing compounds from mast cells. It also blocks IgE antibodies, which cause severe allergic reactions. A good product is Luteolin Complex, made by Swanson Health Products, which contains 100 mg per capsule.

> ➡ **What to do:** Take one to two capsules of Luteolin Complex, three times a day with meals.

▶ Apigenin

This is a flavonoid found in high concentrations in celery, parsley, and apples. It works in a number of ways to inhibit allergic reactions. A good product is Apigenin, made by Swanson Health Products, which contains 50 mg per capsule.

> ➡ **What to do:** Take one 50-mg capsule, three times a day with meals. For more severe allergic reactions, increase each dose to two or three capsules.

▶ Curcumin

A number of studies have shown that curcumin, an extract from the curry spice turmeric, can reduce inflammation and powerfully inhibit allergic reactions. It may even reduce symptoms of first-time occurrences of very severe attacks. CurcumaSorb, made by Pure Encapsulations, contains 250 mg per capsule and is a well-absorbed product.

➤ **What to do:** Take one capsule of CurcumaSorb, three times a day with meals. For more serious allergic reactions, increase each dose to two capsules.

▶ Hesperidin

This is a flavonoid found in high concentrations in oranges. It calms inflammation and reduces allergic reactions and anxiety.

➤ **What to do:** Take 250 mg, three times a day with meals. For more serious allergic reactions, increase each does to 500 mg.

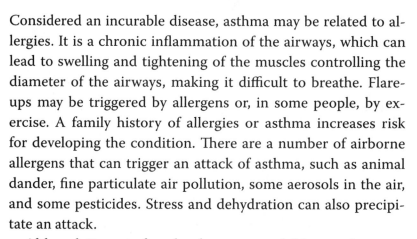

Asthma

Considered an incurable disease, asthma may be related to allergies. It is a chronic inflammation of the airways, which can lead to swelling and tightening of the muscles controlling the diameter of the airways, making it difficult to breathe. Flare-ups may be triggered by allergens or, in some people, by exercise. A family history of allergies or asthma increases risk for developing the condition. There are a number of airborne allergens that can trigger an attack of asthma, such as animal dander, fine particulate air pollution, some aerosols in the air, and some pesticides. Stress and dehydration can also precipitate an attack.

Although it most often develops among children, asthma can occur at any time of life and its incidence is increasing among people over the age of 65, when it becomes more dangerous. Among older people, it may also remain undiagnosed, because symptoms may be mistaken for other respiratory diseases that are more prevalent later in life. Chronic asthma can lead to damage to the smaller airway passages, called bronchioles.

⌇ Conventional Treatment

Asthma rescue medications, usually inhalers, are designed to quell a flare-up, and other drugs aim to control symptoms on an ongoing basis. Steroids are one of the main types of drugs used, but longer-term side effects may include higher blood pressure, ulcers, osteoporosis, cancer, muscle atrophy, and damage to connective tissue.

ASTHMA SYMPTOMS
• Trouble breathing
• Chronic cough
• Wheezing
• Tightness or pain in the chest

In children, asthma sometimes goes into remission as they grow, but this is unlikely among older adults. In addition, people in middle age or later are likely taking other medications, which increases the likelihood of dangerous drug interactions and side effects.

👍 My Recommendations

Food allergies can precipitate asthma-like reactions in some people. Testing for food allergies and intolerances is critical.

Hydration with water is particularly important, as one of the leading causes of asthma attacks is dehydration. Avoid sweetened drinks, as both sugar and aspartame in diet or sugar-free drinks can increase inflammation and worsen asthma. Aspartame, in artificial, zero-calorie sweeteners, is an excitotoxin, as is glutamate in MSG and other food additives commonly found in junk foods (see chapter 2 for a more detailed explanation and list of food additives). Foods naturally high in glutamate may also cause problems and include red meats, soy products (especially soy sauce), tomato sauces, cheeses, and mushrooms.

Natural supplements can help calm inflammation in asthma and reduce allergic reactions that underlie or contribute to the condition. Some of the same supplements that relieve allergies also help to prevent and calm asthma symptoms, since both involve production of irritating histamine and antibodies.

🦌 Natural Supplements

▶ Magnesium

Magnesium reduces inflammation and respiratory symptoms, and protects against blood vessel damage. I recommend taking a malate citrate form, ideally a slow-release magnesium malate called Magnesium w/SRT, made by Jigsaw Health.

➡ **What to do:** Ongoing, take two slow-release tablets of Magnesium w/SRT, twice a day with food. To calm more severe symptoms, use a magnesium citrate or malate product in capsules, which is not slow-release. Empty the contents of four capsules into 6 ounces of water, stir well, and drink.

▶ Vitamin D3

Women deficient in vitamin D3 during pregnancy are more likely to have children who will develop asthma during the first 10 years of life. Other studies have shown that vitamin D3, but not other forms of vitamin D, can reduce inflammation within the small airways (bronchioles) of those with asthma and is especially beneficial if blood levels of vitamin D3 are very low (less than 10 ng/ml).

➡ **What to do:** Get blood levels of vitamin D tested by your doctor and supplement based on individual needs. The optimum level is between 65 ng/ml and 95 ng/ml. Above 100 ng/ml can cause some degree of immune suppression. The dose needed depends on the degree of deficiency.

If the level is less than 30 ng/ml, the dose is 10,000 IU of vitamin D3 a day, taken with a meal, for three weeks, and then repeat the blood test. Once blood levels are in the target range, reduce the daily dose to 5,000 IU.

If the blood level is between 35 and 50 ng/ml, I recommend taking 5,000 IU a day for three weeks and then repeating the blood test. If levels are within the optimum range, reduce the dose to 2,000 IU a day. Babies can take 1,000 IU a day and toddlers and small children can take 2,000 IU a day.

During pregnancy, the mother's dose should be 5,000 IU per day with meals. Infants can take 1,000 IU a day and small children can take 2,000 IU a day.

▶ Vitamin C

High-dose vitamin C reduces inflammatory reactions and can be a great help with asthma. For best absorption, use Lypo-Spheric Vitamin C, made by LivOn Labs, which contains 1,000 mg of vitamin C in one single-serve packet of a gel which gets mixed with water or juice. It works especially well when combined with quercetin (see below). Always take vitamin C without food, as it increases iron absorption, which can lead to iron overload.

> ■ **What to do:** Take one packet of Lypo-Spheric Vitamin C, three times a day without food. For more severe symptoms, take two packets (2,000 mg of vitamin C), three times a day on an empty stomach.

▶ Quercetin

Quercetin is one of the most common flavonoids, a very beneficial category of nutrients found in edible plants. Multiple studies have demonstrated that it has powerful anti-allergy effects, which can help to reduce asthma symptoms. Use a well-absorbed form called Quercenase, made by Thorne Research.

> ■ **What to do:** Take one capsule of Quercenase, three times a day with meals. For more severe symptoms, increase each dose to two capsules.

▶ Luteolin

This is a flavonoid found in high concentrations in celery and artichoke. Multiple studies have shown that it powerfully inhibits the release of histamine and blocks IgE antibodies, both of which play major roles in asthma attacks. A good product is Luteolin Complex, made by Swanson Health Products, which contains 100 mg per capsule.

➡ **What to do:** Take one to two capsules of Luteolin Complex, three times a day with meals.

▶ Apigenin

This is a flavonoid found in high concentrations in celery, parsley, and apples. It works in a number of ways to inhibit allergic reactions involved in asthma. A good product is Apigenin, made by Swanson Health Products, which contains 50 mg per capsule.

➡ **What to do:** Take one 50-mg capsule, three times a day with meals. For more severe symptoms, increase each dose to two or three capsules.

▶ Curcumin

A number of studies have shown that curcumin, an extract from the curry spice turmeric, can reduce inflammation and powerfully inhibit production of antibodies that trigger asthma. CurcumaSorb, made by Pure Encapsulations, contains 250 mg per capsule and is a well-absorbed product.

➡ **What to do:** Take one capsule of CurcumaSorb, three times a day with meals. For more severe symptoms, increase each dose to two capsules.

▶ Hesperidin

This is a flavonoid found in high concentrations in oranges. It calms inflammation and reduces allergic reactions and anxiety.

➡ **What to do:** Take 250 mg, three times a day with meals. For more severe symptoms, increase each dose to 500 mg.

Bronchitis

Bronchitis is a persistent cough, which can be acute, lasting 10 to 20 days or more, or chronic. In both cases, the bronchial tubes, which carry air to the lungs, are inflamed and unable to transport sufficient air or to clear particulate matter and mucus. Most often, acute bronchitis develops as a result of an infection from a cold or flu and lasts longer than the original illness. Exposure to environmental irritants, such as cigarette smoke or other airborne toxins, can also trigger acute bronchitis.

> **BRONCHITIS SYMPTOMS**
>
> - Wheezing
> - Squeaky or whistling sounds when breathing
> - Tightness in the chest
> - Pain in the chest
> - Low fever
> - Shortness of breath, especially when being more physically active
> - Coughing up mucus

Chronic bronchitis is most associated with cigarette smoking. Over time, it causes permanent damage to the lungs and may develop into chronic obstructive pulmonary disease, commonly called COPD. For more details, see the section "COPD." The chronic irritation and inflammation in the bronchial airways increases risk for pneumonia and lung cancer.

🔵 Conventional Treatment

When a cold or flu triggers acute bronchitis, it is a viral infection which can't be treated with antibiotics. In the minority of cases where a bacterial infection is diagnosed, antibiotics are usually prescribed to eradicate the infection. However, repeated or longer-term doses of antibiotics result in disruption of the beneficial bacteria in the colon, which can lead to other serious problems (see "Diarrhea" in chapter 9, "Digestion"). Prescription inhalers are the most common type of medication for symptom relief, and other medications may also be prescribed.

👍 My Recommendations

I have found that a large percentage of people with chronic bronchitis have severe deficiencies in vitamin D3 and vitamin C. Both chronic inflammation and smoking causes a dramatic loss of vitamin C and, to be corrected, requires much larger doses of vitamin C than normal. Nutrient-dense vegetables supply vitamins and other plant compounds that reduce inflammation, fight infections, strengthen connective tissue, and promote healing of damaged tissues. See chapter 3 for how to easily increase your intake with a vegetable drink.

To ease bronchial irritation, use a high-quality air purifier in your home. Also, avoid indoor use of insecticides, commercial bug-control services that use chemicals, and herbicides and pesticides in your yard. These chemicals can impair immunity, worsen lung damage, aggravate inflammation, and increase the risk of developing lung cancer.

🐇 Natural Supplements

▶ Vitamin D3

Studies show that vitamin D3, but not other forms of vitamin D, can reduce inflammation within the small airways, and levels of the vitamin are often low in people with bronchitis.

> ➡ **What to do:** Get blood levels of vitamin D tested by your doctor, and supplement based on individual needs. The optimum level is between 65 ng/ml and 95 ng/ml. Blood levels higher than 100 ng/ml can cause some degree of immune suppression. The dose needed depends on the degree of deficiency.
>
> If your blood level is below 30 ng/ml, I suggest taking 10,000 IU of vitamin D3 daily for one month and then repeating the blood test. If you are in the normal range at that point, cut back the dose to 2,000 IU to 5,000 IU a day. If your blood level is between 30 to 50 ng/ml, I would take 2,000 IU a day with a meal.

▶ Vitamin C

Most people with chronic bronchitis are deficient in vitamin C. It has powerful antiviral and antibacterial properties, strengthens bronchial and lung tissues, reduces inflammation, and neutralizes many free radicals, which can cause serious damage to tissues. For best absorption, use Lypo-Spheric Vitamin C, made by LivOn Labs, which contains 1,000 mg of vitamin C in one single-serve packet of a gel which gets mixed with water or juice.

> ▶ **What to do:** When symptoms are worst, take two to three packets of Lypo-Spheric Vitamin C (2,000 to 3,000 mg of vitamin C), three times a day, especially during flu season. For health maintenance, take one packet (1,000 mg), two to three times a day. Always take vitamin C without food, as it increases iron absorption, which can lead to iron overload.

▶ Mixed Tocopherols and Tocotrienols (Vitamin E)

Although it's usual to hear of "vitamin E" as though it were one single compound, in nature, it's actually made up of multiple nutrients, which fall into the categories of tocopherols and tocotrienols. Usually available as separate supplements—mixed tocopherols and mixed tocotrienols—they should be taken together. They provide powerful protection against a number of harmful substances within the lungs and bronchial tubes and are most effective against ozone, a major atmospheric pollutant.

> ▶ **What to do:** For less severe cases, take 400 IU of mixed tocopherols and 50 mg of mixed tocotrienols, twice a day with meals. For more severe cases, double each dose.

▶ N-Acetyl Cysteine (NAC)

NAC is a compound that safely increases cellular levels of glutathione, a major internal antioxidant in our bodies, which counteracts damaging free radicals and lipid peroxidation. It reduces the thickness of mucus, protects lung tissue, and helps relieve bronchitis symptoms.

➡ **What to do:** Take 500 to 750 mg, once a day with a full meal. It should never be taken on an empty stomach as it can cause severe cramping. Should you develop stomach cramping, for quick relief, take two capsules of DGL plus, made by Pure Encapsulations. (It also relieves heartburn.)

▶ Hyperbaric Oxygen Therapy (HBOT)

I am not aware of any studies of HBOT as a treatment for bronchitis. However, since this is an inflammatory disorder triggered by infection, and HBOT reduces inflammation and infection, it should improve the severity of bronchitis and reduce the incidence of episodes.

Chronic Obstructive Pulmonary Disease (COPD)

COPD is a combination of lung disorders, most often chronic bronchitis and emphysema, which make it difficult to breathe. Each disorder impairs breathing in a slightly different way: chronic bronchitis inflames, irritates, and blocks the bronchial tubes that transport air to lungs. Emphysema involves the air sacs themselves.

In the deepest part of the lungs, there are tiny air sacs which take in oxygen and eliminate waste, such as carbon dioxide. The exchange occurs through the membranes of the sacs. In healthy lungs, these sacs are very small, allowing a great number to be packed into the lungs, and this maximizes the surface area through which oxygen and other gases can move in and out of the lungs. When emphysema develops, the number of sacs decreases and the remaining ones become bigger, reducing the overall surface area. As a result, the lungs cannot take in as much oxygen or eliminate as much carbon dioxide,and breathing becomes progressively more difficult.

Overall, 20 percent of people who smoke for some time will develop COPD, and 50 percent of lifelong smokers will develope the disorder. Air pollution is responsible for acute worsening of the condition. The use of sewage sludge for landfill contributes heavily to this problem, as the dust from these contaminated soils (called biosolids) contains toxic metals and highly immune-stimulating particulate matter that significantly worsens bronchial and lung irritation and inflammation. Even public parks use these highly contaminated soils.

> **SIGNS OF COPD**
>
> One or more of these may indicate COPD or a greater risk for the disease:
>
> - Difficulty breathing, especially after physical exertion
> - Breathing becomes more difficult over time
> - A persistent cough
> - Chronic production of mucus, or sputum, in the chest
> - Being a smoker
> - Ongoing exposure to dust, smoke, or chemicals that emit airborne toxins
> - A family history of lung disease

Conventional Treatment

Most COPD is caused by long-term smoking, and quitting is essential. Recurrent, severe pulmonary infections are common and can make the condition advance much more rapidly. Prescription inhalers and oral medications are designed to open up bronchial tubes, and steroids may be prescribed to reduce inflammation, but there is no cure. Many people with COPD are continually on oxygen therapy. In some cases, surgery is done to remove damaged lung tissue that impairs breathing and, in extreme cases, lung transplants may be done, but are accompanied by high risks.

My Recommendations

As with bronchitis, it is important to remove as many lung irritants as possible, such as smoking and ambient air pollution.

High-quality air filters should be used in the home, especially in the bedroom. The best ones also filter out chemical pollutants. In addition, remove mold pollution from your house, especially black mold, and do not use insecticides in your home or pesticides or herbicides in your yard.

Diet can play a major role in improving COPD. Replace inflammatory fats, such as corn, safflower, sunflower, peanut, soybean, and canola oils with coconut oil or extra virgin olive oil; use anti-inflammatory herbs in food, such as turmeric or rosemary; and cut back on sugar, which can significantly increase inflammation and hence lung damage. Skip beef and eat no more than 6 ounces a day of poultry or pork. Eat plenty of vegetables and have a vegetable drink at least once a day, per my recipe in chapter 3. Vegetables contain high levels of magnesium, which helps to calm overly reactive bronchial tissues.

Iron should not be taken in supplements, unless medically supervised as a result of documented iron deficiency.

Natural Supplements

▶ Vitamin C

Vitamin C levels are generally low in smokers and people with COPD and need to be corrected with high doses of vitamin C supplements. It reduces inflammation and promotes healing of damaged tissues. I recommend a high-absorption form, Lypo-Spheric Vitamin C, made by LivOn Labs, which contains 1,000 mg of vitamin C in one single-serve packet of a gel form.

- ➡ **What to do:** For milder symptoms, I recommend one packet (1,000 mg of vitamin C) mixed with 4 ounces of juice or water, two or three times a day between meals. For severe symptoms, you can increase the dose to two to three packets (2,000 mg to 3,000 mg), three times a day, always between meals.

▶ **Vitamin D3**

Vitamin D3 is an immune modulator, meaning it keeps the immune system balanced, and it reduces inflammation and kills viruses and bacteria. All these effects help to reduce COPD symptoms.

➡ **What to do:** Get blood levels of vitamin D tested by your doctor and supplement based on individual needs. The optimum level is between 65 ng/ml and 95 ng/ml. Blood levels higher than 100 ng/ml can cause some degree of immune suppression. The dose needed depends on the degree of deficiency.

If your blood level is below 30 ng/ml, I suggest taking 10,000 IU of vitamin D3 daily for one month, and then repeating the blood test. If you are in the normal range at that point, cut back the dose to 2,000 to 5,000 IU a day. If your blood level is between 30 to 50 ng/ml, I would take 2,000 IU a day with a meal.

▶ **Multivitamin/Mineral**

Chronic inflammatory diseases cause a general depletion of many vitamins and minerals, many needed for reducing inflammation and repairing damaged tissue. The product should include mixed carotenoids and a variety of B-vitamins. If you are eating 10 servings of nutrient-dense vegetables a day, a multivitamin and mineral supplement can be overlooked.

➡ **What to do:** Take a balanced multivitamin and mineral supplement daily, such as Extend Core, made by Vitamin Research Products. Take two capsules of Extend Core, three times a day, with meals.

▶ **Mixed Tocopherols and Tocotrienols (Vitamin E)**

Although it's usual to hear of "vitamin E" as though it were one single compound, in nature, it's actually made up of multiple nutrients, which fall into the categories of tocopherols and tocotrienols. Usually available as separate supplements—mixed tocopherols and mixed tocotrienols—they should be taken together. They provide powerful protection against a number of harmful substances within the lungs and bronchial tubes and are most effective against ozone, a major atmospheric pollutant.

> ➡ **What to do:** For less severe cases, take 400 IU of mixed tocopherols and 50 mg of mixed tocotrienols, twice a day with meals. For more severe cases, double each dose.

▶ Curcumin

Animal studies have found that curcumin is powerful in protecting bronchial tissues and air sacs within lungs against damage caused by smoking, air pollution, and infection. Some studies have also shown that it prevented changes that lead to cancer, a high risk with COPD. Curcumin fights inflammation, viruses, and bacteria, and promotes healing of damaged bronchial and lung tissues. CurcumaSorb, made by Pure Encapsulations, contains 250 mg per capsule and is a well-absorbed product.

> ➡ **What to do:** Take one capsule of CurcumaSorb, three times a day with meals. For more severe symptoms, increase each dose to two capsules.

▶ Quercetin

Quercetin has anti-inflammatory, antiviral, antioxidant, and cancer-inhibiting properties. Studies have shown that it reduces airway inflammation and improves elasticity of bronchial tissues, which enables better air exchange. Use a well-absorbed form called Quercenase, made by Thorne Research.

> ➡ **What to do:** Take one capsule of Quercenase (250 mg of quercetin), three times a day with meals. For more severe symptoms, increase each dose to two capsules.

▶ Resveratrol

This substance is found in grape skins in high concentrations. Several studies have shown that it provides benefits for those suffering from COPD and other pulmonary diseases, because it has powerful antioxidant and anti-inflammatory properties. In lab research, resveratrol protected human lung cells against damage from cigarette smoke. It should be taken with niacinamide (vitamin B3).

➡ **What to do:** Take 200 mg of resveratrol with 250 mg of niacinamide, twice a day with meals.

▶ Baicalin

An extract from the skullcap plant, baicalin has anti-inflammatory, antioxidant, antianxiety, anticancer, and brain-protective effects. Recent animal studies have shown that it significantly protects against smoking-induced damage. I recommend using a powdered version simply called Baicalin, made by LiftMode.

➡ **What to do:** Mix one-half teaspoon of baicalin powder with a teaspoon of extra virgin olive oil and take this mixture three times a day, with meals.

▶ Hyperbaric Oxygen Therapy (HBOT)

With COPD, there is inflammation and poor oxygenation of tissues—characteristics that HBOT is known to improve. Therefore, HBOT should provide some relief from COPD symptoms.

Colds and Flu

Colds and flu are viral infections, with different viruses, and the flu is more serious than a cold. While not all symptoms are the same, some overlap and can make it difficult to tell the two infections apart. For elderly people and anyone with a compromised immune system, the flu can be dangerous because it can lead to pneumonia or other life-threatening conditions.

However, a commonly cited statistic that 36,000 people die of the flu each year is pure fiction created by flu vaccine proponents.

In most years, only a few hundred die of actual flu, most of whom have significant health conditions that lower resistance and immunity. Many listed as dying of the flu in fact die from other conditions, such as asthma or heart failure. The most common cause of death in those infected with the influenza virus is not caused by the virus itself but rather from a person's excessive immune reaction to the virus, called a "cytokine storm." A number of nutritional extracts can prevent and stop this deadly reaction.

Conventional Treatment

Many people mistakenly ask their doctor for (and receive) antibiotics, which work only for bacterial infections. Since colds and flu are viral, antibiotics can't help, and taking them unnecessarily contributes to antibiotic resistance, which can be dangerous if a real bacterial infection needs to be treated in the future. In addition, several types of antibiotics, such as tetracyclines, can suppress the most important type of antiviral immunity, called cellular immunity. Cholesterol-lowering statin drugs are also powerful immune suppressants and can increase the incidence and severity of colds and flu.

Over-the-counter decongestants and fever-suppressing drugs are the most common conventional treatments. In some cases, doctors may prescribe antiviral drugs. There are no medications to prevent colds or flu, other than flu vaccines, which pose other risks and are not always effective.

COLD OR FLU?

A sore throat, runny nose, congested nasal passages, and a cough can be symptoms of either a cold or flu, but beyond that, these are some ways to tell them apart:

- A cold generally lasts no more than a week, whereas the flu can last longer and is more severe.

- Fever, headache, and overall muscle aches are typically signs of the flu, although milder versions of these may accompany a cold.

- With a cold, a fever is more likely to occur among young children.

- A feeling of exhaustion is more likely and more severe at the onset of the flu, but can occur to a lesser degree with a cold.

Prevention by vaccines is a hit and miss proposition, as in many years the wrong virus is anticipated.

Lowering one's temperature with drugs, such as ibuprofen and aspirin, can actually worsen the infection and its complications, especially in young children. In fact, lowering fever in small children has been shown to dramatically increase mortality from viral infections, because viruses do not tolerate high temperatures and a fever is a natural way to fight them.

Drugs such as ibuprofen and aspirin can relieve an achy feeling, but they also reduce your immune system's ability to heal, which prolongs the infection. The achy feeling is not caused by the virus but rather by your immune reaction to the virus.

👍 My Recommendations

To protect yourself against colds and flu, the most important thing you can do is to build a healthy immune system. Foods that help to do this also reduce inflammation in the diet I describe in chapter 1. In a nutshell, it includes a lot of vegetables, especially organic ones, some meat, filtered water, and healthy fats such as extra virgin olive oil and coconut oil. Onion, garlic, and many spices, such as oregano, sage, and turmeric, the curry spice, have antiviral qualities.

Immune-suppressing foods and ingredients include trans fats, sugar, high-starch carbohydrates, grains, cow's milk, processed foods, and food additives with glutamate, such as MSG and others listed in chapter 2. Fluoride, mercury, cadmium, lead, pesticides, herbicides, and fungicides all suppress or disrupt immunity and should be avoided.

🐇 Natural Supplements
▶ Beta Glucan

Technically called beta-1,3/1,6-glucan, this is an extract from the cell walls of baker's yeast. When highly purified, it can improve the efficiency of cell-mediated immunity, your most important antiviral defense system. (By the way, this type of immune function is not activated by vaccination.) I usually take beta glucan when I know I will be exposed to infected people or will be traveling on airplanes, buses, or trains. It is most effective in preventing infections or when taken at the first sign of illness.

➤ **What to do:** Take 500 mg on an empty stomach and do not eat anything for at least 30 minutes afterward. This dose can be repeated daily for three days and then reduced to 250 mg a day, until you are well or no longer exposed to infected people. During flu season, especially when it is at its height in your area, take 500 mg at least once a week. Anyone with an autoimmune disease should work with a physician who is knowledgeable about beta glucan to avoid overstimulating the immune system.

▶ **Vitamin C**

If taken in a highly absorbable form, vitamin C has powerful antiviral characteristics and effectively reduces the immune system's reaction to infection with a virus (the cytokine storm). Lypo-Spheric Vitamin C, made by LivOn Labs, which contains 1,000 mg of vitamin C in one single-serve packet of a gel form, is a highly absorbable, effective product.

➤ **What to do:** If you feel cold or flu symptoms coming on, take two packets (2,000 mg of vitamin C), mixed with water or juice, three times a day on an empty stomach, until the illness passes. For prevention, take one packet (1,000 mg of vitamin C) mixed with 4 ounces of juice or water, two or three times a day between meals.

▶ **Curcumin**

An extract of the curry spice turmeric, curcumin has powerful antiviral properties, reduces inflammation, and prevents damage that is a byproduct of the immune system fighting viruses, but not all curcumin is well absorbed. CurcumaSorb, made by Pure

Encapsulations, contains 250 mg per capsule and is a well-absorbed, effective product.

> ➠ **What to do:** Take one capsule of CurcumaSorb, three times a day with meals.

▶ Quercetin

Quercetin is one of the most commonly found flavonoids, therapeutic compounds found in vegetables, teas, and fruits. A recent study found that it is a powerful inhibitor of cold viruses. Quercetin also works in another way, by helping to reduce excess iron, which is used by a virus to replicate itself. The quercetin binds with excess iron, making it unavailable to a virus. Use a well-absorbed form called Quercenase, made by Thorne Research.

> ➠ **What to do:** Take one capsule of Quercenase (250 mg of quercetin), three times a day with meals.

▶ N-Acetyl Cysteine (NAC)

NAC is a compound that safely increases cellular levels of glutathione, a major internal antioxidant in our bodies, which protects cells and tissues from damage by free radicals and lipid peroxidation products. Studies have shown that NAC can shorten the course of flu infections and colds.

> ➠ **What to do:** Take 500 to 750 mg, once a day with a full meal. It should never be taken on an empty stomach as it can cause severe cramping. Should you develop stomach cramping, for quick relief, take two capsules of DGL plus (which also relieves heartburn), made by Pure Encapsulations.

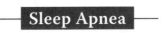

Sleep Apnea

In Greek, *apnea* means "without breath." In the case of sleep apnea, a person's breathing stops during sleep, most often because certain muscles, which surround the airway and control breathing, relax to

RISK FOR SLEEP APNEA

The condition is twice as common in men, compared to women, and its likelihood increases with:

- Obesity
- Being middle-aged or older
- Sedative drugs
- Alcohol
- A relatively large tongue
- A relatively small throat
- A large neck size

a point of blocking the passage of air. This can happen 30 or more times per hour and is called obstructive sleep apnea. A common cause of snoring, mostly among men, it not only interferes with restful sleep, but also increases risks for memory problems, high blood pressure, diabetes, heart disease, stroke, depression, and accidents that occur as a result of drowsiness during the day.

Less often, breathing can be interrupted because of a malfunction in brain signals related to breathing. Called central sleep apnea, this condition doesn't cause snoring and is likely a side effect of a separate medical condition or medication, which should be treated as needed.

Conventional Treatment

For obstructive sleep apnea, the most common type, diagnosis is the first step. Often, a family member or the person's bed partner is the one to notice signs of the condition. A complete diagnosis includes a sleep study in a lab or having a person use a device that tracks sleep patterns at home.

Treatment may include weight loss, sleeping in a different position, reducing the use of sedative drugs or alcohol, or wearing a dental device at night to reposition the jaw and parts of the mouth. Or, a continuous positive airway pressure (CPAP) machine may be recommended. It uses air pressure to prevent blockage during sleep and is considered the most effective treatment. In rare cases, surgery may be recommended, but is risky.

My Recommendations

Newer research shows that inflammation is intimately related to sleep apnea and may originate from fat inside the abdomen. This special fat releases inflammatory substances called cytokines, which in turn affect the breathing centers within the brain stem. In a study of obese individuals, surgical removal of abdominal fat cured a high percentage of people with sleep apnea. It is unknown why only a select few will develop sleep apnea, given the widespread incidence of inflammation and obesity.

The most important thing one can do is reduce excessive abdominal fat, also called a pot belly, and lower levels of chronic inflammation. chapters 1 through 3 describe the way to do it, and the "Obesity" section, in chapter 14, "Chronic Conditions," explains more about the link to inflammation.

Natural Supplements

▶ Resveratrol

Found in higher concentrations in grape skins, resveratrol reduces the effect of abdominal fat on inflammation and protects the brain.

> ⇒ **What to do:** Take 200 mg, once or twice a day with a meal, depending on the severity of the problem.

▶ Curcumin

Curcumin is a powerful antioxidant and anti-inflammatory. Studies have shown that it can reduce inflammation as efficiently as corticosteroids, without the side effects. However, it is important to take a highly absorbable form, such as CurcumaSorb, made by Pure Encapsulations. It contains 250 mg per capsule.

> ⇒ **What to do:** Take two capsules, two to three times a day with meals.

▶ Quercetin

Quercetin inhibits inflammation through a different process than curcumin, so by taking both, one gets maximum benefits. Quercenase, made by Thorne Research, is particularly well absorbed. Each capsule contains 250 mg.

> ⇒ **What to do:** Take one capsule, three times a day with meals.

▶ Luteolin

This naturally occurring flavonoid, a type of beneficial plant compound, reduces inflammation connected with sleep apnea. It suppresses two major types of cells, macrophages and microglia, which drive the inflammation.

➡ **What to do:** Take 100 mg, three times a day, and gradually increase each dose to 300 mg. It is best taken with food.

▶ Apigenin

Like luteolin, apigenin suppresses the same types of drivers of inflammation related to sleep apnea. However, each plant extract works slightly differently, so the two are complementary. Apigenin, made by Swanson Health Products, contains 50 mg per capsule.

➡ **What to do:** Start by taking two capsules, three times a day with food. This can be increased to four capsules, three times a day, as needed.

▶ Lypo-Spheric Vitamin C

Vitamin C can calm some underlying mechanisms of the nervous system that are involved in sleep apnea. Lypo-Spheric Vitamin C, made by LivOn Labs, is combined with a phospholipid, a waxy substance naturally present in our bodies, which makes it absorbable and easy on the digestive system. It comes in packets of a gel, which gets mixed with water or juice. Each packet contains 1,000 mg of vitamin C.

➡ **What to do:** Mix one packet with 4 ounces of water or juice and take this three times a day on an empty stomach. Do not take vitamin C with food, as it increases absorption of iron, which can lead to excessive iron intake.

▶ Mixed Tocopherols and Tocotrienols (Vitamin E)

Natural vitamin E is not a single nutrient but is made up of eight forms. These fall within two major groups, called tocopherols and tocotrienols. In combination, they offer powerful protection against an internal process akin to rusting.

➡ **What to do:** Take 400 IU of mixed tocopherols and 100 mg of mixed tocotrienols, once or twice a day.

▶ Multivitamin/Mineral

A good multivitamin and mineral supplement should include all of the B vitamins, carotenoids, zinc, selenium, and no iron.

➡ **What to do:** Take per product directions.

▶ Hyperbaric Oxygen Therapy (HBOT)

Most sleep apnea is caused by an excess of deep abdominal fat, which releases powerful inflammatory chemicals that cause the telltale breathing problems. Losing this particular type of fat reduces symptoms or eliminates the disorder. Since HBOT has been shown to reduce both inflammation and obesity, it increases the chances of a cure.

CHAPTER 14

Chronic Conditions

Cholesterol and Heart Attacks

Cholesterol has long been touted as the leading cause of heart attacks by being the major culprit in atherosclerosis, but this isn't actually the case. Compelling evidence shows that oxidation of a number of oils, including cholesterol, is the driving mechanism for atherosclerosis. With atherosclerosis, plaque builds up in arteries and interferes with blood flow to our organs and tissues. The plaque is made up of inflammatory fats, cholesterol, numerous white blood cells, calcium, and other substances found in blood. Hardened plaque narrows arteries and, by limiting the flow of oxygen and nutrients, damages the heart, brain, and other organs. Plaque affects large and small blood vessels. Ruptured plaque, which results in the formation of a blood clot, may cause a total blockage and trigger a heart attack.

Careful studies have shown that the buildup of fatty streaks, the precursor to plaque, begins to develop in childhood and advances considerably by age 20. One study found that 17 percent of teenagers had some degree of atherosclerosis, and after age 50 it was present in 85 percent of people, even though it did not affect health and function equally among individuals. While death rates as a result of heart attacks have been falling, the incidence of atherosclerosis has not. Heart attacks and strokes combined remain the leading killer in the United States and many other industrialized nations.

WAYS TO PREVENT PLAQUE
Although plaque naturally builds up with age, these are some ways to reduce it:
• Not smoking
• Eating plenty of fruits and vegetables
• Controlling weight, especially around the belly
• Reducing stress
• Limiting or avoiding alcohol
• Exercising regularly
• Avoiding inflammatory fats
• Increasing intake of anti-inflammatory fats, such as omega-3 oil in fish
• Regularly brushing and flossing teeth
• Avoiding exposure to fluoride
• Avoiding exposure to toxic metals, such as aluminum, cadmium, or lead
• Avoiding food additives with glutamate, such as MSG

The latest research now shows that the main culprit behind atherosclerosis is chronic inflammation within the inner lining of the arteries. The cause of this inflammation varies considerably, and in most instances there are a number of causes interacting. For example, all these cause inflammation: chronic bacterial or viral infections; exposure to toxic metals, such as lead, mercury, cadmium, or aluminum; a poor diet; stress; high blood pressure; environmental pollutants such as exhaust fumes; and autoimmune diseases.

Conventional Treatment

The common wisdom is that elevated cholesterol is a major contributor to the buildup of plaque, but this idea is not supported by scientific evidence. Nevertheless, prescriptions for cholesterol drugs are commonplace and, among older people, are often part of a combination of medications which can lead to debilitating side effects, including disorientation, memory loss, muscle weakness, and death.

Careful studies have shown that after age 65, statin drugs have no effect on heart attacks and can worsen health. Compared to younger people, older individuals require higher cholesterol levels for good health, especially brain health. In addition, statins are potent immune-suppressing drugs and can increase the risk of cancers and infections.

In cases of dangerous arterial blockages, stents or bypass surgery are accepted treatments by orthodox medicine. Stents have not been as successful as expected, since arteries treated with stents usually become blocked again within three to five years.

👍 My Recommendations

In reducing atherosclerosis, the goal is to reduce inflammation. Diet, which is most critical, and anti-inflammatory supplements offer the best course to achieve this goal. See chapter 1 for the anti-inflammatory diet and lifestyle in more detail, but these are the key points:

- Eat and drink vegetables (recipe is in chapter 3)
- Eat the right meats
- Know your fats
- Drink purified water and white and green teas
- Avoid trans fats
- Avoid sugar
- Minimize carbohydrates
- Avoid fluoride

- Maintain healthy teeth
- Exercise regularly
- Avoid prolonged, excessive stress

What most people find surprising is that sugar, so copious in today's food supply, is the big driver of atherosclerosis and heart disease. Despite what your doctor may tell you, saturated fat is not the bad guy. While I'm not advocating overindulgence in fatty foods, I can't emphasize enough that sugar is the culprit, and it has many variations.

High fructose corn syrup, for example, is in just about any kind of packaged or processed food. It's found in soups, sauces, savory breads and buns, condiments, frozen meals, processed meats, and many "healthy" foods, such as flavored yogurts. Because this sweetener has been criticized, some food products are now touted for containing "real cane sugar." This is still sugar, and it doesn't make such foods any healthier. An overabundance of starch has the same effect, because starch is turned into sugar in the human body.

🐇 Natural Supplements

As well as eating an anti-inflammatory diet, it is important to take a multivitamin for essential vitamins and minerals. In addition, many plant extracts and nutrient compounds have very powerful anti-inflammatory and antioxidant properties that reduce atherosclerosis. These are some of the best ones.

▶ Curcumin

Studies show that curcumin, an extract from the curry spice turmeric, is one of the most powerful anti-inflammatory compounds and can dramatically reduce atherosclerosis. And, it has a slight anticoagulant effect, which helps reduce heart attacks. CurcumaSorb, made by Pure Encapsulations, contains 250 mg per capsule and is a well-absorbed product.

➧ **What to do:** Take one to two capsules of CurcumaSorb, three times a day with meals.

▶ Quercetin

Another powerful anti-inflammatory and antioxidant, in animal studies, quercetin has produced significant improvements in severe atherosclerosis. Use a well-absorbed product such as Quercenase, made by Thorne Research.

➧ **What to do:** Take one capsule of Quercenase, which contains 250 mg of quercetin, three times a day with meals.

▶ Luteolin

Several studies have shown that Luteolin inhibits atherosclerosis through a number of mechanisms. It calms special white blood cells, called macrophages, which play a major role in atherosclerosis. A good product is Luteolin Complex, made by Swanson Health Products, which contains 100 mg per capsule.

➧ **What to do:** Take two capsules of Luteolin Complex, three times a day with meals.

▶ Apigenin

Found in celery, parsley, and apples, it is a powerful anti-inflammatory and inhibits atherosclerosis. A good product is Apigenin, made by Swanson Health Products, which contains 50 mg per capsule.

➧ **What to do:** Take two capsules, three times a day with meals

▶ Aged Garlic Extract

This is a special form of garlic. A number of human studies have shown that it not only reduces atherosclerosis, but might reverse it as well. The product, which is odorless, is called Kyolic Aged Garlic Extract, made by Wakunaga.

➧ **What to do:** Take one capsule of Kyolic Aged Garlic Extract 100% Vegetarian Cardiovascular Formula 100, twice a day with meals.

▶ **Mixed Tocopherols and Tocotrienols (Vitamin E)**

Natural vitamin E is not one single compound but a combination, grouped into subtypes called tocopherols and tocotrienols. Together, they offer rather powerful inhibition of atherosclerosis.

➡ **What to do:** Take 400 IU of mixed tocopherols and 50 mg of mixed tocotrienols, twice a day, with or without meals.

▶ **Magnesium**

Magnesium reduces inflammation, raises levels of our major internal antioxidant, glutathione, helps to keep arteries flexible, and improves blood flow, even through the smallest blood vessels, called arterioles and capillaries. For optimum absorption, take either magnesium citrate or malate. A slow-release form is best, such as Magnesium w/SRT, made by Jigsaw Health.

➡ **What to do:** Take two slow-release tablets, twice a day with meals.

▶ **Hyperbaric Oxygen Therapy (HBOT)**

At least one animal study found that HBOT could reduce atherosclerosis. This makes sense, as HBOT reduces inflammation within the walls of blood vessels, and such inflammation leads to atherosclerosis.

Diabetes, Type 2

Marked by elevated levels of blood sugar, type 2 diabetes is the most common form of the disease. Its incidence is growing at unprecedented levels, as levels of obesity, lack of physical activity, and a poor diet become more prevalent.

The disease develops when there is a malfunction in insulin, the hormone that gets blood sugar into cells, where it can be used to generate energy. With type 2 diabetes, the cells are unable to take in the blood sugar, and levels in the blood become chronically elevated. This impairment is also described as insulin resistance, because the cells are literally resistant to the normal function of insulin.

> **SYMPTOMS OF TYPE-2 DIABETES**
>
> Signs of type 2 diabetes include:
> - Being hungry after eating
> - Feeling tired
> - Being very thirsty
> - Urinating often
> - Losing weight without reason
> - Numbness in the hands or feet
> - Blurry vision
> - Sores that heal very slowly

Over a period of time, the high blood sugar damages blood vessels and leads to heart disease, deterioration of vision, kidney damage, impotence, and damage to nerves in the extremities of the body. Type 2 diabetes is also associated with degeneration of the brain, which can lead to memory loss, disorientation, confusion, and poor attention. Strokes and heart attacks are much more common in people with type 2 diabetes.

Conventional Treatment

Type 2 diabetes is an incurable disease, according to conventional medicine, but most cases can be prevented, and many can be reversed with the right lifestyle. Weight loss, where necessary, regular exercise, and a healthy diet are the most important factors. However, medications to lower levels of blood sugar are the most common treatment, largely because most physicians are not trained to help patients effectively change their lifestyles. Over time, a body's ability to produce insulin may also deteriorate, and at that point, insulin shots become necessary.

My Recommendations

Diet and exercise are most important in preventing and reversing this condition. There is compelling evidence that the typical Western diet is playing a key role in type 2 diabetes, mainly because of the massive intake of sugar and starch, as well as the consumption of inflammatory omega-6 oils and trans-fats. High fructose corn syrup is a big enemy, as it can worsen the damage caused by diabetes. Exposure to MSG early in life can result in lifelong insulin resistance that leads to type 2 diabetes.

Diet should be anti-inflammatory, as described in chapter 1. It should include a few carbohydrates with each meal but should be limited in quantity, such as one slice of bread a day. Avoid diet foods and beverages with aspartame, as it is carcinogenic, damages the brain, and worsens atherosclerosis. I also discourage soy products, as they are high in manganese, fluoride, aluminum, and glutamate, all of which can make diabetics worse.

Exercise is critical, especially muscle-building resistance exercises. It improves uptake of glucose by muscles, thereby lowering harmful levels of glucose in the blood. Exercise also reduces atherosclerosis, which is very aggressive in diabetics, and improves blood flow through the smaller blood vessels.

Natural Supplements

One of the interesting characteristics of flavonoids, therapeutic components of plants, is that most stimulate insulin function, thereby improving glucose entry into cells and overcoming insulin resistance that underlies diabetes. In addition, most also reduce inflammation and are powerful antioxidants, and these characteristics reduce complications of diabetes, such as blindness, strokes, heart attacks, peripheral vascular disease, and nerve damage.

Natural supplements work best when following a good diet and a regular exercise program. While there are a number of flavonoid supplements that can help diabetes, these are the safest and most reliable.

▶ Cinnamon Extract

A relative of the turmeric plant, cinnamon has been shown to significantly improve insulin function and lower elevated blood sugar. It also reduces inflammation.

➡ **What to do:** It is important to use a pure cinnamon extract and not cinnamon bark. For benefits, the dose varies widely, from 1,000 to 6,000 mg a day.

▶ R-Lipoic Acid

This extract is a natural substance found in all cells and tissues and is one of the most important and powerful antioxidants. It also lowers elevated blood sugar and improves insulin resistance. It is a form of alpha-lipoic acid, but the R form is much more powerful.

➡ **What to do:** Take between 300 and 600 mg with each meal.

▶ Curcumin

A recent study found that curcumin can not only prevent diabetes from occurring, but can also greatly improve elevated blood sugar and correct insulin resistance. In addition, it can prevent, to a large extent, the atherosclerosis buildup associated with diabetes. The best form to take is CurcumaSorb, made by Pure Encapsulations, which contains 250 mg per capsule and is a well absorbed product.

➡ **What to do:** Two capsules, which contain 500 mg, with each meal will have a maximum effect. Safety for much higher doses of curcumin has been established.

▶ Multivitamin/Mineral

I recommend a well-balanced multivitamin and mineral supplement. The B vitamins, when possible, should be in their most functional form. Specifically, folic acid or folate should be in the form of MTHF, short for 5-methyltetrahydrofolate; vitamin B6 should be in the form of pyridoxal 5-phosphate; and riboflavin (vitamin B2) in the form of riboflavin 5'-phosphate. These forms are much more effective for diabetes. Basic Nutrients V, made by Thorne Research, is an example of such a product.

➡ **What to do:** Take a multivitamin with the recommended forms of B vitamins, per product directions.

▶ Hyperbaric Oxygen Therapy (HBOT)

HBOT has been shown to improve insulin resistance, the cause of type 2 diabetes. In addition, it can reduce the risk of complications by helping to reverse two other harmful aspects of diabetes: widespread inflammation and a destruction of small blood vessels.

Fatigue

A symptom that may be a side effect of many medical conditions or prescription drugs, fatigue can also be a manifestation of poor nutrition, lack of restful sleep due to pain or bad sleep habits, lack of exercise, depression, or stressful situations in life. It could also be a reaction to one or more food additives or toxins in the environment, or a combination of these. By itself, it has no simple medical diagnosis, but diet and lifestyle issues are often an underlying factor, one that is not likely to be addressed in routine medical care, but can be remedied by taking charge of one's health in everyday life.

One basic aspect of fatigue is an impaired ability of the cells to generate sufficient energy. Within cells, 95 percent of all energy is produced by parts of a cell called mitochondria. Infections and environmental toxins, such as toxic metals, industrial chemicals, pesticides, herbicides, and fungicides, can interfere with mitochondrial energy production.

WHY EXERCISE REDUCES FATIGUE

Studies show that gentle exercise, as little as a 15-minute walk, increases energy and reduces fatigue in many cases. One analysis, which looked at 70 studies with more than 6,800 people, found that exercise consistently boosts energy, and it doesn't need to be extremely demanding. The effect of exercise was, on average greater than that of stimulant medications, and helped both healthy people and those receiving treatment for serious diseases, such as diabetes, heart disease, and cancer. It's possible that exercise may enhance energy and relieve fatigue by working on the central nervous system.

Conventional Treatment

Because fatigue can be a sign of many other conditions, or can stem from a lack of proper nutrition, medicine has no protocol for identifying what's wrong or how to remedy the situation by looking solely at fatigue. A medical diagnosis would begin with an inventory of risk factors, other symptoms, a medical history, and possibly customized testing, depending on the individual's situation. All too often, women who complain of fatigue but don't have an obvious underlying condition are misdiagnosed as being depressed and are prescribed antidepressants. These neither address nor resolve the problem and can lead to further deterioration as a result of side effects.

My Recommendations

Improving diet can reduce or even cure fatigue. In practice, that means following the anti-inflammatory diet I've described in chapter 1. Over the years, this is what I have consistently noticed: when people switch from their usual Western diet to the anti-inflammatory diet for just two weeks, they all return saying that they have more energy than they had even as a youth. When moderate exercise is added, they experience even greater energy.

Why are the benefits so dramatic? The Western diet, high in sugar, starch, and unhealthy fats, is a prescription for fatigue, because it is the perfect diet for generating inflammatory chemicals within the human body. These impair mitochondria, the energy-production components of every cell, and lack of energy is an inevitable result.

Natural Supplements

In severe cases of fatigue, especially when related to diseases, one may require an additional boost of cellular energy production. Many plant extracts and nutrients enhance energy but they also need to efficiently mop up waste products. The ones below are some of the best at performing both functions.

▶ Coenzyme Q10 (CoQ10)

This is a substance that is naturally present in our bodies, but levels decline as we age. It is critical for energy production by mitochondria, and is an antioxidant. Statin drugs are notorious for depleting CoQ10 and, as a result, causing severe fatigue. Studies have shown that supplemental CoQ10 improves energy production and can even dramatically improve chronic fatigue syndrome.

➡ **What to do:** The dose varies with the severity of fatigue. In most cases, a dose of 125 to 250 mg, three times a day with meals will suffice. Higher doses, such as 500 to several thousand mg can be used but are quite expensive. The most easily absorbed CoQ10 is suspended in an oil or is in a "nanosized" form.

▶ Niacinamide

Another name for vitamin B3, niacinamide is essential for production of a critical energy molecule. It does not cause any flushing effect, as niacin does, and poses no risks.

➡ **What to do:** The usual dose is 500 mg, taken two to three times a day with meals. It can be dissolved in water but has a strong, bitter taste.

▶ Riboflavin 5'-Phosphate (R-5-P)

This is a form of riboflavin (vitamin B2), which is used by cells during energy production. With age, we lose some of the ability to generate the R-5-P form of the vitamin, but supplements can solve the problem. Many products contain only very small amounts but R-5-P, made by Swanson Health Products, contains 50 mg per capsule.

➡ **What to do:** Take 50 mg, once or twice a day with meals.

▶ Pyridoxal 5-Phosphate (P-5-P)

This is the form of vitamin B6 used by cells to make energy. Another form of B6, pyridoxine, can damage nerves if taken in very high doses (much higher than I'm recommending). However, P-5-P has never been shown to cause a problem, even when the dose is several thousand milligrams.

➡ **What to do:** Take 50 mg of P-5-P per day, in the morning with a meal.

▶ Methylcobalamin (vitamin B12)

Vitamin B12 comes in more than one form. Methylcobalamin is the one for boosting energy production, and it is very well absorbed.

➡ **What to do:** Take 500 mcg or more per day, depending upon your personal response.

▶ Carnitine and R-Lipoic Acid

A natural energy molecule used by all cells, carnitine can be found in supplements as L-carnitine or acetyl-L-carnitine, which is more expensive but also beneficial for the brain. Both increase energy, so either form can be taken. Along with carnitine, I recommend taking R-lipoic acid, an antioxidant, to mop up waste products from the process of generating additional energy.

➡ **What to do:** Take 250 to 500 mg of carnitine and 100 mg of R-lipoic acid, three times a day with meals.

▶ Magnesium Malate

A specific form of magnesium, this plays a vital role in hundreds of reactions involved in energy generation, mops up waste products, and reduces inflammation. For best absorption, I recommend a slow-release form, such as Magnesium w/ SRT, made by Jigsaw Health.

➡ **What to do:** Take two slow-release tablets, twice a day with meals.

▶ Zinc Picolinate

Zinc is essential for more than 300 biochemical reactions in the body, many of which produce energy. Zinc deficiency is very common with chronic diseases, aging, and fatigue.

➡ **What to do:** Take 30 mg, three times a week.

▶ Hyperbaric Oxygen Therapy (HBOT)

Research has shown that HBOT can reduce fatigue. In some studies, it even improved symptoms in people suffering from chronic fatigue syndrome.

High Blood Pressure

As blood circulates, it exerts force against the walls of the arteries. Blood pressure is a measurement of that force. Arteries have a layer of muscle that contracts and relaxes to control blood pressure and flow, which is essential for delivering oxygen and nutrients to tissues and organs. Sometimes, the walls of arteries become stiff, with atherosclerosis, for example, and this raises blood pressure. High blood pressure, or hypertension, raises risk for heart attacks, strokes, kidney damage, accelerated brain aging, and early death. Because it typically has no visible signs or symptoms, it's often called the "silent killer."

Doctors use two numbers to measure blood pressure. As an example, these are written as 120/80 or spoken as "120 over 80." This is what the numbers mean:

The top number: Indicates the amount of force each time your heart beats, and is called systolic blood pressure.

The bottom number: Indicates the amount of pressure that remains inside the arteries each time your heart rests in between beats, and is called diastolic blood pressure. Stiff arteries are a major cause of high diastolic blood pressure.

Optimum blood pressure: This is 120/80. Medically speaking, 140/90 is called "first stage hypertension," but some studies suggest that health risk begins to increase at lower levels that are above 120/80. Other studies find no real problems as long as systolic blood pressure (the top number) is below 140. The higher the numbers, the greater the risk. However, elderly people have less elastic arteries and require higher blood pressure, around 140 systolic, to maintain blood flow to their vital organs, such as kidneys, heart, and brain.

Conventional Treatment

Lifestyle changes are the first and most important step for prevention and treatment. These

> ### SIDE EFFECTS OF DRUGS THAT LOWER BLOOD PRESSURE
>
> Side effects discourage many people from taking these medications. They include:
> - Erectile dysfunction
> - Loss of libido among men and women
> - Fatigue, which can be extreme
> - Nausea
> - Heartburn
> - Difficulty swallowing
> - Damage to the heart muscle
> - Shortness of breath
> - Dizziness
> - Flu-like symptoms
> - Irregular heart beat (arrhythmia)
> - Depression
> - Disorientation
> - Memory loss
> - Liver failure
> - Swelling that looks similar to hives (angioedema)

include losing weight (especially abdominal fat) where necessary, becoming more physically active, eating less sugar, eating more vegetables and some fruit, drinking only in moderation, and not smoking. When this approach isn't enough, or isn't followed, there are more than 50 prescription drugs that can lower blood pressure by working in a variety of ways. For example, some regulate the muscle within the walls of arteries, while others relax the heart, and often, doctors prescribe a combination. These medications have many complications, including fatigue and, in men, impotence, which explains why so many stop taking their medications.

👍 My Recommendations

Medicine classifies 90 percent of high blood pressure as "essential hypertension," meaning it has no known cause. Inflammation is the triggering mechanism in most cases. Over many years, arterial inflammation damages the walls of blood vessels and makes them stiffer, which raises blood pressure.

Regular exercise, such as walking 30 minutes daily, and the right diet are the starting point. For anyone who is overweight, losing weight is key, but rather than focusing on the scale, start by changing eating habits, mainly removing sugar, processed foods, fruits juices, and particularly breads from your diet. Newer research shows that previous ideas about salt elevating blood pressure were in error and that the real culprit all along was sugar.

Dairy products—which doctors routinely recommend for lowering blood pressure—can be problematic because many people don't digest them well. Some studies have shown a dramatic increase in heart attacks and strokes in those consuming the most dairy products, and unless these are organic, they are a source of synthetic hormones, antibiotics, and pesticides, which are all detrimental.

I recommend following the anti-inflammatory diet in chapter 1. These are the key points:

- Eat five to ten servings of high-nutrient vegetables each day.

- Have a vegetable drink every day, using my recipe in chapter 3.

- Avoid dairy products.

- Consume more anti-inflammatory omega-3 oils in fish and avoid inflammatory vegetable oils.

- Avoid food additives that are excitotoxins, such as MSG and aspartame in artificial sweeteners (see chapter 2 for more details).

• Get fiber from vegetables and legumes, rather than grains.

• Avoid all sugar.

• Drink water that is filtered and free of fluoride, cadmium, lead, and aluminum.

If you do this and still have elevated blood pressure, add supplements.

Natural Supplements

In combination with weight loss, regular exercise, and dietary changes, specific supplements can be much more effective than drugs in treating hypertension. They create virtually no side effects and offer additional benefits.

If you are currently taking blood-pressure medication or other drugs for a heart condition or diabetes, you will need to work with a doctor who is educated in natural medicine. This is especially important with hawthorn, as it increases the toxicity of some drugs.

▶ Hawthorn

Hawthorn extract is accepted by many cardiologists to be as effective as powerful medications. But unlike drugs, it enhances heart health in more ways than one, and its efficacy is supported by extensive lab and human testing.

Hawthorn relaxes blood vessels and reduces fatty substances that slow down blood flow. And, it strengthens heart muscle contractions, thereby enhancing the flow of blood through key arteries connected to the heart, kidneys, and brain. The herb also contains antioxidants and fights bacteria, and these properties help to keep the heart and blood vessels in shape.

The benefits of hawthorn are greater when it's taken along with a balanced multivitamin, such as Extend Core, made by Vitamin Research Products, and the other nutrients below.

However, if you were to choose only one natural supplement for high blood pressure, hawthorn would be the logical choice.

▶ **What to do:** To lower blood pressure, take 200 to 500 mg, three times daily. Start with the lower dose and gradually increase it. To prevent hypertension, start with 100 mg, two or three times daily. If you are taking medications, use hawthorn under the guidance of a doctor.

▶ Curcumin and Quercetin

Both of these flavonoids, therapeutic compounds in plants, have been shown to lower severe hypertension in animal studies. The mechanism involves their anti-inflammatory effects. In the case of curcumin, it has an ability to increase nitric oxide, which relaxes arteries and restores healthy function of the artery lining. They also protect all the organs affected by hypertension, including the heart, kidneys, and brain. Curcumin specifically reduces hypertension caused by exposure to cadmium. Curcumin should be taken as CurcumaSorb, made by Pure Encapsulations, and quercetin as Quercenase, made by Thorne Research.

▶ **What to do:** Take 500 mg of CurcumaSorb, and 250 mg of Quercenase, three times a day with meals.

▶ Hesperidin Methyl Chalcone

This is a special form of hesperidin, found in citrus fruits. It protects and strengthens blood vessels and helps them to dilate more easily.

▶ **What to do:** Take between 500 and 1,000 mg, three times a day with meals.

▶ DHA

One of the major components of fish oil, DHA (short for docosahexaenoic acid) reduces blood pressure, improves blood flow, corrects damage to the heart, and improves overall health. DHA powerfully reduces inflammation throughout the body and in blood vessels.

➡ **What to do:** Take 1,000 to 1,200 mg daily with a meal.

▶ Aged Garlic Extract

An odorless, concentrated form of garlic, it lowers blood pressure, protects the heart, and improves overall health. It also fights infections, which can cause hypertension and damage arteries. The product is called Kyolic Aged Garlic Extract, made by Wakunaga.

➡ **What to do:** Take 600 mgs once or twice daily with food.

▶ Coenzyme Q10 (CoQ10)

In studies, CoQ10 has lowered blood pressure in people with hypertension, diabetes, and heart disease. In one study of 83 people, the supplement lowered blood pressure better than a combination of prescription drugs. Many blood-pressure-lowering drugs and cholesterol-lowering statin drugs deplete CoQ10, and this contributes to side effects and deterioration of the heart. People who take CoQ10 often report having more energy.

➡ **What to do:** Take 125 to 600 mg, one to three times daily with food, depending upon your response. "Nanosized" CoQ10 or CoQ10 in an oil improves absorption.

▶ Carnitine

Some studies, though not all, have found that carnitine, also called L-carnitine, lowers blood pressure. In addition, research shows that it can relieve weakness that is a side effect of blood-pressure-lowering drugs. Acetyl-L-carnitine, a form that is also good for the brain, is also beneficial for lowering hypertension.

➡ **What to do:** Take 500 mg, two to three times daily, on an empty stomach.

▶ N-Acetyl-L-Cysteine (NAC)

The supplement has reduced blood pressure in animal research and is especially good for hypertensive people who are at risk for diabetes or have the disease. NAC reduces the effects of stress on blood pressure. Never take NAC on an empty stomach as it can cause severe cramping. NAC increases the level of glutathione, a critical internal antioxidant made by our bodies.

➡ **What to do:** Take 500 to 1,000 mg daily, immediately after a full meal.

▶ Alpha-Lipoic Acid

A natural antioxidant found in every cell, the supplement should be taken by anyone who has hypertension plus diabetes or is at risk for the disease.

➡ **What to do:** Take 50 mg, just before your largest meal of the day. If you have type 2 diabetes, take a form of the nutrient known as R-lipoic acid. Start with 100 mg, three times daily, 30 minutes before each meal, and gradually increase the dose in 50-mg increments, until your blood sugar reaches a healthy level.

Insomnia

Insomnia is difficulty falling or staying asleep, assuming one has allowed enough time to get a good night's rest. It can occur occasionally, for days or weeks, or can be chronic. In chronic cases, the insomnia is usually a symptom of some other problem, such as a medical condition or a side effect of medications. Insomnia can lead to weight gain and obesity, irritability, inability to concentrate, memory problems, anxiety, depression, slow reaction times, and increased risk for developing chronic diseases such as diabetes.

💊 Conventional Treatment

All too often, doctors prescribe sleeping pills, which can create a dependence and dangerous side effects, including daytime drowsiness, which can contribute to falls or other accidents. Some sleep prescriptions can result in sleepwalking and even homicidal and suicidal tendencies. Among older people who take multiple prescriptions, interactions can cause insomnia. A complete evaluation would include a review of drugs and possible undiagnosed medical conditions. In addition, sleep studies can be done, either in a medical center or with a device an individual wears at home, to track sleep patterns during the night.

👍 My Recommendations

An inflammatory diet, low-grade infections, and gum infections as a result of poor dental hygiene can all contribute to insomnia by causing chronic inflammation. A blood test, called high sensitivity C-reactive protein, or hs-CRP for short, measures levels of chronic inflammation. However, it's always advisable to eat an anti-inflammatory diet, described in chapter 1.

While exercise is one of the ways to reduce inflammation, it's best to do it before 6 pm. Later, especially if it is intense, exercise can make it difficult to fall asleep. Demanding mental activities before bedtime also lead to wakefulness, including reading a serious non-fiction book, doing one's taxes, using electronic devices, and marital squabbling.

Helpful bedtime routines include reading relaxing fiction and, for some

> **COMMON TRIGGERS OF INSOMNIA**
>
> In addition to medical conditions and prescription drugs, sleep can be disrupted by:
> - Shift work
> - Travel through different time zones
> - An underactive or overactive thyroid
> - Hormonal changes before and during menopause, or during menstrual cycles
> - Caffeine, alcohol, and other stimulants
> - Use of electronic devices before bedtime
> - Having some light in the bedroom

people, listening to soft music. During the night, the room should be completely dark and quiet.

These are some other causes of insomnia that are often overlooked:

Nighttime hypoglycemia: Blood sugar falls too low during the night and this activates the brain, leading to full wakefulness. It is a common cause of awakening during the middle of the night. To prevent it, eat your evening meal later, even as late as 9 pm, but avoid desserts, sweet drinks, alcohol, and starchy foods, as these can overstimulate the brain. As an alternative, snack on a small amount of meat, such as turkey, and a few cashew nuts, about an hour before bed.

Glutamate: Food additives with glutamate, such as MSG, described in chapter 2, are powerful brain activators and can cause severe insomnia. And some foods are high in glutamate. One of the characteristics is forced thinking, where thoughts are flying through your mind like a film on fast-forward. Insomnia is only one of many reasons to avoid glutamate.

Low melatonin: Our levels of this natural sleep hormone tend to decrease with chronic illness and aging, making it difficult to get to sleep. Aspartame in chemical zero-calorie sweeteners and fluoride interfere with its production and should be avoided.

Natural Supplements

Taking magnesium and calcium at bedtime helps to induce sleep, and there are various sleep formulas of plant extracts and nutrients which you can try. I've found the ones below to be particularly effective, without causing addiction, dependence, or side effects.

▶ Melatonin

This is a hormone manufactured by the brain (by the pineal gland). The level naturally rises just before bedtime and falls when we are about to awaken in the morning. Light, even in small amounts, can rapidly shut down its production. Melatonin not only helps us sleep, but is also one of the brain's most powerful antioxidants, and protects the entire body. Taking melatonin supplements will not interfere with our natural ability to produce the hormone.

➡ **What to do:** The dose needed can vary. I suggest starting with no more than 0.5 mg, taken 30 minutes before bedtime. This will work for most people, but if it doesn't, you can try a higher dose. Taking too much can sometimes interfere with sleep. I recommend a sublingual form, which dissolves under the tongue. If you wake up during the night, don't turn on any bright lights, take another 0.5 mg, and lie quietly in bed. Even if you cannot fall asleep, remain in bed, lie very still, and relax, rather than trying to plan the next day or solve problems. Studies have shown that even though you feel fully awake, you are getting important rest.

▶ Hesperidin Methyl Chalcone

This is a specific form of hesperidin, found in high concentrations in oranges, which has been shown to calm the brain and improve sleep. I have used it in patients with insomnia with good results, enabling very restful sleep. However, in people who suffer from reactive hypoglycemia, a condition in which blood sugar drops very low within a few hours after eating, the supplements can have an opposite effect, waking them up.

➡ **What to do:** Take 250 mg 30 minutes before bedtime.

Obesity

Obesity isn't the same as simply being overweight. It means having too much body fat, to a point where health risks significantly increase, with higher likelihood of heart disease, stroke, diabetes, some cancers, and arthritis. As the numbers of obese

FAT FACT

Most of us have known obese people who lived to a ripe old age—but not many. Newer research shows that the location of fat, rather than obesity itself, is the real culprit in increasing risk for diseases and death.

Abdominal fat—around the intestines, inside the abdomen—and not the fat under the skin, appears to be the bad guy. This special fat releases high levels of very harmful inflammatory compounds called cytokines. These inflammatory chemicals lead to a host of deadly conditions, such as atherosclerosis, cancer, diabetes, strokes, liver failure, hypertension, sleep apnea, and kidney damage.

Studies in people have shown when this abdominal fat is surgically removed, blood pressure returns to normal, type 2 diabetes subsides, sleep apnea disappears, and underlying risk factors for heart disease and diabetes improve. However, removing superficial fat under the skin has no beneficial effects.

Interestingly, a person can appear relatively thin and still have excess abdominal fat, so conventional measures of body weight, which do not take this into account, can be deceptive. Weight loss that targets the inflammatory abdominal fat is very beneficial.

people have increased in recent decades, the medical community has not been able to find a way to solve the problem. Although new weight-loss drugs have been developed over the years, they have had minor success, and some have been withdrawn due to dangerous side effects.

Conventional Treatment

In recent years, surgery to force a person to eat less has been gaining popularity. There are basically two types, both limiting the size of the stomach, leading to a feeling of fullness after eating less food. One type, which is reversible, is the insertion of a laparoscopic band to limit expansion of the stomach. For ongoing weight loss, the band needs to be adjusted from time to time, to continue decreasing the size of the stomach. The other type, which is not reversible, surgically seals off or removes part of the stomach, making it permanently smaller.

After both types of surgery, patients need to make lifestyle changes to learn how to continually eat more nutritious food in smaller quantities, and to become more active. With the more extreme, permanent type of surgery, there can be dangerous nutrient absorption problems, and diet needs to be controlled to ensure enough vitamins and minerals. In addition, many people just eat more often, even though their stomachs are smaller, and continue to consume large amounts of sugar and starch calories—the ones that cause health problems.

👍 My Recommendations

There are a great number of diets and diet books. Although many (but not all) contain some good information, no diet is worthwhile if you cannot stick to it—forever! And severe low-calorie diets cause loss of muscle tissue and can lead to weakness and heart damage.

In the 1970s, Dr. Atkins demonstrated to the medical community that eating fat has nothing to do with getting fat; it was all due to sugar and carbohydrates. Since then, many others have proven this premise, finding that the leading cause of obesity is an excess of sugar and starchy carbohydrates, which leads to high levels of blood sugar, excessive release of insulin, deposition of deep fat in the abdominal area, and chronic inflammation.

Although you can't "spot reduce" when trying to lose weight, eating sugars and starches in excessive amounts, so common today, produces the opposite effect: somewhat selective fat gain, most often called "belly fat." Although the location of fat is not limited to the belly, it deposits there to a harmful and usually noticeable degree. Cutting out the sugars and starches, along with some moderate exercise and high-nutrient foods, will eventually shrink a belly and the health risks that go along with it.

The diet I recommend, in chapter 1, eliminates the major bad foods—the breads, buns, crackers, chips, pretzels, and cereals that all make you gain fat—and the massive amounts of sugar Americans now consume, especially in sodas and other sweetened drinks. These provoke considerable insulin release and fat deposition—especially abdominal fat.

Another major cause of the so-called obesity epidemic is massive consumption of foods with glutamate additives, such as MSG (monosodium glutamate) under many different names on food labels (see chapter 2). A great number of studies have shown that feeding MSG to baby animals causes them to become grossly obese early in life, and to remain obese. They also quickly develop the precursors of diabetes. And, this obesity is very resistant to dieting and exercise.

Natural Supplements

While there are a number of supplements available for fat loss, in general, I do not recommend any of them. The most commonly promoted weight-loss products today include guarana, green coffee bean extract, and raspberry ketones. In most cases, those selling such extracts emphasize the need for a controlled diet and regular exercise. And most contain higher concentrations of stimulants such as caffeine, which can stress the brain and heart, resulting in long-term damage.

Other products combine green tea extract with caffeine and other metabolic boosters, which can produce fat loss, but can also harm the brain and increase the production of harmful free radicals. Green tea has not been shown to result in fat loss except in certain animal studies using very high concentrations of an extract.

I prefer a common-sense program of controlling insulin- stimulating foods mentioned above, and regular exercise. Chapter 1 describes it in more detail.

▶ Safe Natural Sugar Substitutes

I generally recommend avoiding all artificial sweeteners, such as aspartame, Neotame, acesulfame K, and sucralose (in Splenda). All have been shown to have harmful effects and some, such as aspartame, can induce several cancers in laboratory animals. Likewise, sugar alcohols, such as erythritrol, isomalt, maltitol, mannitol, sorbitol, and xylitol, all have health issues. Xylitol has been shown to cause brain damage in higher concentrations. Some others can cause severe diarrhea in some people.

The only sweeteners that have pretty safe records include stevia and a product called Just Like Sugar®, which is made from orange peel and chicory root, and contains some calcium and vitamin C. Stevia, in those with reactive hypoglycemia, a disorder of very low blood-sugar levels, can cause a precipitous fall in blood sugar.

▶ **Hyperbaric Oxygen Therapy (HBOT)**
Several studies have shown that HBOT can reduce obesity. This is an important benefit, since weight loss is difficult for most people, yet obesity is associated with elevated levels of inflammation throughout the body and many chronic, debilitating conditions.

Osteoarthritis

The most common type of arthritis, osteoarthritis causes joint pain and stiffness. It doesn't necessarily affect the same joints on both sides of the body. Those most commonly affected are the knees, hips, neck, lower back, thumbs, fingers, in the joints closest to the nails. Its key characteristic is a degeneration of cartilage in joints.

Cartilage is hard but slippery tissue that acts as a cushion in the joint, absorbs shock from movement, and allows bones to glide painlessly as the joint moves. With osteoarthritis, some of the cartilage wears away, narrowing the

RISK FOR OSTEOARTHRITIS

Although the incidence of osteoarthritis increases with age, it can also occur in younger people as a result of joint injury. This is especially true for high-stress joints such as the knees. Throughout life, these increase risk:

- Being overweight, which puts added stress on joints
- Injuries that damage cartilage and other tissue that cushions joints
- Lack of physical activity
- A diet that includes inflammatory foods

normal space between bones and allowing them to rub together, and this causes pain, stiffness, and swelling. Small pieces of cartilage or bone, which can break off and float in the joint space, can cause more pain.

In the past, osteoarthritis was considered a non-inflammatory form of arthritis, but recent research shows that it is, in fact, inflammatory, but of a much lower intensity than, say, rheumatoid arthritis. This indolent inflammation weakens the cartilage, resulting in a slow erosion, leaving the joint without its natural protection. Repeated trauma to a joint can trigger the inflammatory process.

Conventional Treatment

Medications to control pain are a major conventional treatment for osteoarthritis, but risks of side effects increase with longer-term use, and drugs do not heal degenerated cartilage or other tissue. When pain and impaired function is severe, joint replacement surgery is often indicated. In recent years, exercise is more frequently recommended, as studies have shown that it reduces pain, increases mobility, and enhances an individual's overall quality of life. Exercise in water is often a starting point because it is the most gentle on joints.

Because of the discovery that osteoarthritis is an inflammatory disease, newer drugs are being designed to reduce inflammation. The present anti-inflammatory drugs have far too many complications for long-term use. For example, the COX-2 blocking drugs, Bextra and Vioxx, were withdrawn from the market as a result of deaths from heart attacks. Another one, Celebrex, is still used but carries warnings about increasing risk of heart attacks and strokes that can lead to death.

My Recommendations

Diet is very important as it can either reduce or worsen inflammation. The typical Western diet, high in inflammatory vegetable oils, sugar, red meats, and dairy products, worsens inflammation and weakens joints. Preferably, meats should be eaten only once or twice a week, but if eaten daily, the quantity should be no more than 6 ounces. The better meats include chicken, turkey, duck, and seafood (I consider fish a meat). At least five to ten servings of vegetables should be eaten with a minimal amount of fruits. Blended vegetable drinks, as in my recipe in chapter 3, are easier to absorb than solid raw vegetables and help meet dietary goals.

To calm osteoarthritis, avoid all fluoride-containing products and fluoridated drinking water, as fluoride causes bone destruction and an overgrowth of bone spurs. Fluoride is found in toothpaste, mouthwash, dental treatments, black tea, and many medications, both over-the-counter and prescription.

Resistance exercises strengthen ligaments, tendons, and muscles and improves bone strength, all of which helps to protect joints. However, avoid using weights that are too heavy and stress joints. Water exercises are gentle on joints.

Natural Supplements

The goal of supplements is to reduce inflammation and enhance the rebuilding of joint cartilage. While there are many supplements people use to treat osteoarthritis, the following are, in my experience, the most useful and safest.

▶ Curcumin and Quercetin

The combination of these two flavonoids, therapeutic components of plants, makes up some of the most powerful anti-inflammatory substances available, equal to prescription drugs, but without the terrible side effects. In the human body, there are multiple mechanisms of inflammation. This natural duo is so successful because it reduces all types of these, whereas drugs address only one mechanism. For curcumin, a well-absorbed form is CurcumaSorb, made by Pure Encapsulations, and for quercetin, Quercenase, made by Thorne Research.

➡ **What to do:** Take 250 to 500 mg of CurcumaSorb, two to three times a day with meals, depending on the severity of the problem. As well, take 250 mg of Quercenase, three times a day with meals.

▶ MSM (Methylsulfonylmethane)

A type of sulfur found in plants and animals, MSM has a long history of effectively reducing inflammation and pain, especially in joints.

➡ **What to do:** Take 850 mg, three times a day with food until the pain subsides, and then once a day for maintenance.

▶ Chondroitin Sulfate and Glucosamine

These two compounds are major components of connective tissues and cartilage. They are best for chronic joint conditions, especially osteoarthritis, but have also been useful in rheumatoid arthritis.

➡ **What to do:** Take 500 mg of glucosamine and 250 mg of chondroitin, three times a day.

▶ BioCell Collagen

Collagen is the "glue" that holds tissue together and is a key component of healthy joints. BioCell Collagen is a particular form of collagen which, in studies, has been shown to reduce joint destruction in a number of joint diseases, including osteoarthritis and rheumatoid arthritis. One good product is Collagen JS, made by Pure Encapsulations, which contains 1,000 mg of BioCell Collagen in two capsules.

➡ **What to do:** Take two to four capsules of Collagen JS a day, with meals.

▶ Hyperbaric Oxygen Therapy (HBOT)

Inflammation perpetuates pain and stiffness in osteoarthritis and HBOT reduces inflammation. Some studies have shown that HBOT reduces joint pain.

Osteoporosis

Although women are more prone to this disorder, older men also face a significant risk of osteoporosis. The word literally means "porous bones," which become weak, brittle, and more likely to break, even with little or no external force. Bones are living tissue and are continually breaking down and being rebuilt. When osteoporosis develops, there is an imbalance among these two actions, where too much bone is lost and not enough is restored. Although bone mass in the human body reaches its peak in the 20s, and then gradually declines, osteoporosis is not a natural or inevitable part of aging.

Conventional Treatment

Different drugs may be prescribed, depending on an individual's situation. The most popular ones are in a category called bisphosphonates, such as Fosamax. Widely advertised, these slow the cycle of bone breakdown, resulting in a modest increase in bone mass. However, bone produced while taking such drugs is more brittle and may increase risk for some types of fractures. Side effects may include heartburn, throat pain, chest pain, abnormal heart rhythm, swallowing difficulties, and other pain. In some cases, the drugs prevent bone in the jaw from healing after a tooth extraction or other dental surgery, which can be a serious problem that leads to loss of bone in the jaw.

My Recommendations

Most problems with bone density are due to two main events: a diet that makes the body too acidic and a lack of resistance exercise.

Our activity influences what happens in our bones. When we

> **WHAT INCREASES RISK FOR OSTEOPOROSIS?**
>
> Some risk factors cannot be changed, such as getting older, having a family history of osteoporosis, or being a woman, especially a small-boned, thin one. But these are risk factors we can control:
>
> - Being physically inactive
> - Following a diet that lacks essential vitamins, minerals, and protein
> - Smoking

lift weights, working arms and legs, ligaments and tendons pull on bones and stimulate them to deposit more calcium. As a result of these exercises, our bones become denser. The opposite is seen when astronauts are in space for extended times. When we first sent men into space for prolonged periods, we discovered that they experienced a tremendous loss of bone calcium and hence bone strength. Because they were in a very low-gravity situation, there was very little force exerted on their bones. Exercise helped reverse this, but not completely.

A diet that makes our bodies too acidic contributes to bone deterioration. Red meat and sugar are highly acidic foods, and should be avoided or limited. Populations that eat a mostly vegetarian diet, which is alkalizing, rarely get osteoporosis, even in old age. An anti-osteoporosis diet should contain at least five to ten servings of vegetables that are high in calcium and magnesium, as the two minerals are more beneficial for bones than calcium alone. Such vegetables include spinach, collard greens, turnip greens, mustard greens, garlic, arugula, broccoli, and okra.

A therapeutic category of nutrients, flavonoids, have also been shown to reduce the risk of osteoporosis. They include naringin, quercetin, silymarin, green tea, curcumin, resveratrol, and hesperidin. Eating a variety of green and highly colored vegetables will supply most of these, and they are available as individual supplements. Hesperidin is especially useful in preventing bone loss in older men.

In addition, fluoride in water, toothpaste, mouthwash, and other products should be avoided, because it is the great destroyer of bones. It was once considered a possible remedy for osteoporosis but was found to increase fracture rates.

Natural Supplements
▶ Calcium
Most people are aware that the strength of bone comes from its calcium content, but less well appreciated, even by many

doctors, is that calcium supplements may not improve calcium deficiencies in bones. This is because not all forms of calcium are well absorbed and utilized by the human body. Tums, for example, contain calcium carbonate, which is not well used by bones, and they contain artificial colors and flavors, which are toxins.

Vegetables can supply most of your calcium, if you eat enough of them. Otherwise, take a supplement of the calcium citrate form, which can be utilized by bones. Or, take calcium pyruvate; pyruvate is another nutrient that protects the brain and heals the gut, and this form of calcium is well absorbed.

➡ **What to do:** Never take more than 500 mg of calcium a day from supplements, as you will always get some from food, and the supplement is only to guard against a shortfall. In men and anyone who has had cancer, too much calcium in supplements can promote cancer growth. Don't take calcium with tap water or any food that may contain aluminum, as calcium increases absorption of the toxic metal.

▶ Magnesium

Magnesium plays an important role in depositing calcium where it needs to be—within the bones. Also, by reducing inflammation, magnesium prevents mineral loss from bones. For best absorption, I prefer a slow-release form of magnesium malate, such as Magnesium w/SRT, made by Jigsaw Health.

➡ **What to do:** Two tablets (250 mg) of Magnesium w/SRT, twice a day, are usually sufficient, especially if one is eating the suggested five to ten servings of vegetables.

▶ Vitamin K

Studies have shown that vitamin K supplementation reduced fractures and prolonged survival in postmenopausal women, especially when taken with calcium and vitamin D3 (see my vitamin D recommendations in chapter 1). A subtype of vitamin

K2, called MK-7 (short for MenaQ7), appears to provide the greatest benefit and is available in many supplements.

> ➡ **What to do:** Take 100 to 200 mcg of MK-7 a day. If you are taking anticoagulant drugs that block vitamin K, notify your doctor first.

▶ Zinc

This is another mineral that plays an important role in bone formation and strength. The picolinate form is recommended.

> ➡ **What to do:** Take 15 mg of zinc picolinate a day.

Rheumatoid Arthritis

Although its cause is unknown, rheumatoid arthritis is recognized as an autoimmune disorder, which means the body's immune system attacks tissue as though it were an invader. Most often, it strikes joints in the fingers, wrists, elbows, shoulders, knees, ankles, and/or feet, usually on both sides of the body. It may begin with stiffness and pain in one joint, and then progress to others. Over time, the disease damages joints and may cause them to become deformed.

Because the inflammation associated with this disorder affects many tissues and organs besides joints, it can cause a host of other serious and even life-endangering problems. These include neurodegeneration, depression, anxiety, muscle atrophy and weakness, heart failure, increased risk of heart attacks and strokes, gut problems, kidney failure, liver damage, and others. There is some evidence that chronic infections with mycoplasma organisms, tiny bacteria that do not respond to many antibiotics, may underlie the triggering of the autoimmune reaction.

Conventional Treatment

There is no cure for rheumatoid arthritis as yet. Unlike osteoarthritis, which affects one or more specific joints, rheumatoid arthritis influences the whole body. Different types of drugs, commonly used in combination, aim to reduce inflammation and suppress the immune system reaction that drives the disease. A more recent treatment is aimed at a single inflammatory cytokine called tumor necrosis alpha (TNF-alpha), which is suppressed by drugs such as etanercept (Enbrel) and infliximab (Remicade). Treatments using a variety of drugs may be given orally, as injections, or intravenously.

SYMPTOMS OF RHEUMATOID ARTHRITIS
In addition to affecting joints, the disease can also produce these symptoms: • Fatigue • Tingling, numbness, or a burning sensation in hands or feet • Dry mouth • Dry eyes • Itching or burning in the eyes • Chest pain when inhaling a breath • Sleep disturbances

In extreme cases, joint surgery may be done to remove damaged tissue or replace a joint. Physical therapy, including heat and cold therapies, and splints to realign and support joints, may also be part of treatment.

👍 My Recommendations

A number of studies have examined dietary treatments and report varying degrees of positive results, with some showing dramatic improvements and others minor improvements. Most such studies do not control for some important factors, for example certain foods that can aggravate inflammation.

In general, red meats and overall high-meat diets worsen symptoms. This may be related to meats having high levels of iron, which can contribute to inflammation, and glutamate (the same ingredient that is in MSG). Glutamate (described in more detail in chapter 2) is what I call an excitotoxin, known to play a major role in inflammation and pain and to cause damage to tissues and organs, including the brain. It is especially important to avoid all processed foods that contain glutamate, which is added to foods only to enhance taste, and overstimulates nerve cells.

In addition, a diet high in the vegetable oils in processed foods, such as corn, sunflower, safflower, peanut, soybean, and canola oils, can greatly worsen inflammation, tissue destruction, and pain. Processed foods should be avoided and these oils should be replaced with coconut oil or extra virgin olive oil, both anti-inflammatory. Extra virgin olive oil also contains a number of powerful antioxidants. Chapter 1 covers this in more detail.

Vegetables contain thousands of anti-inflammatory compounds. Eat at least five servings of fresh, organically grown, nutrient-dense vegetables, such as kale, other greens, celery, parsley, cauliflower, cabbage, onions, and garlic, per day. An easier solution is to make a blended vegetable drink, which greatly increases nutrient absorption and cuts down on the volume of vegetables. A 12-ounce glass of a vegetable blend can contain the equivalent of 10 to 12 servings of raw vegetables eaten whole. My recipe is in chapter 3.

It is also a good idea to have one's stool tested. This will measure bacterial counts and types of organisms in the colon. If yeast is found, it should be treated vigorously as it will worsen the immune attack on joints.

Natural Supplements

▶ Curcumin and Quercetin

These are two of the leading and most powerful anti-inflammatory compounds found in nature. In fact, in combination they are as powerful as steroids, but without the terrible side effects. Because of a relatively short half-life, they should be taken every four to six hours.

➡ **What to do:** Take well-absorbed forms in capsules, such as CurcumaSorb, made by Pure Encapsulations, and Quercenase, made by Thorne Research. Take 500 mg of each, three times a day with meals. If you choose other brands, to enhance absorption, open the capsules and mix capsule contents with coconut oil or extra virgin olive oil. Thoroughly mix one tablespoon of the oil and 500 mg of each supplement, take the mixture, and then have a drink of water.

▶ Apigenin

This naturally occurring plant flavonoid is a powerful anti-inflammatory and especially inhibits the immune cell that is causing most of the trouble in rheumatoid arthritis, the macrophage.

➡ **What to do:** Take two 100-mg capsules, three times a day with meals.

▶ Luteolin

Like apigenin, this plant flavonoid also inhibits the macrophage and is a powerful anti-inflammatory.

➡ **What to do:** Take two 100-mg capsules, three times a day with meals.

▶ More Flavonoids

There are a number of other powerful anti-inflammatory flavonoids that can be added, such as silymarin (which also protects the liver and brain), resveratrol, EGCG from green tea, and naringenin. All are available in supplements and, in combination, have synergistic, beneficial effects. If you blend a vegetable drink as I describe in chapter 3, you can empty the contents of these capsules directly into the blend.

▶ Fish Oil

It contains two main components that reduce inflammation, called EPA and DHA. In severe inflammatory disorders, such as rheumatoid arthritis, it's best to take a mix of the two, which is naturally found in fish oil. One good product is Carlson's Fish Oil, a concentrated, high-dose, liquid form which, for many people, is easier to take than multiple capsules. It comes in two flavors, orange and lemon.

➡ **What to do:** Take two tablespoons, twice a day with meals.

▶ Magnesium and Zinc

Inflammation causes a rapid and extensive loss of magnesium and zinc. The more intense and prolonged the inflammation, the greater the loss of these essential metals. For magnesium, a slow-release form of magnesium malate is best tolerated and is available as Magnesium w/SRT, made by Jigsaw Health. For zinc, take a picolinate form.

> ➡ **What to do:** Take two tablets of Magnesium w/SRT, two to three times a day with meals, and 30 mg a day of zinc picolinate.

▶ Probiotics

Since the colon bacteria play such a vital role in immunity, take a broad-spectrum probiotic, with a combination of beneficial bacteria and some prebiotics, which provide food for the beneficial organisms. One such product is Theralac, made by Master Supplements.

> ➡ **What to do:** Take one capsule of Therelac, at least once or twice a week. If you are taking antibiotics, take two capsules, twice a day until the antibiotic is stopped, and then return to the lower dose.

▶ Chondroitin Sulfate and Glucosamine

These two compounds are major components of connective tissues and cartilage. They are best for chronic joint conditions, especially osteoarthritis, but have also been useful in rheumatoid arthritis.

> ➡ **What to do:** Take 500 mg of glucosamine and 250 mg of chondroitin, three times a day.

▶ BioCell Collagen

Collagen is the "glue" that holds tissue together and is a key component of healthy joints. BioCell Collagen is a particular form of collagen which, in studies, has been shown to reduce joint destruction in a number of joint diseases, including osteoarthritis and rheumatoid arthritis. One good product is Collagen JS, made by Pure Encapsulations, which contains 1,000 mg of Bio-Cell Collagen in two capsules.

➥ **What to do:** Take two to four capsules of Collagen JS a day, with meals.

▶ Hyperbaric Oxygen Therapy (HBOT)

Because of its ability to reduce inflammation, HBOT holds promise in reducing the damage caused by rheumatoid arthritis. It also may reduce symptoms of the disease, such as pain and weakness.

CHAPTER 15

Brain Health

» ADHD

» Alzheimer's,
   Parkinson's, and ALS

» Anxiety

» Brain Aging

» Depression

» Memory Loss,
   Age-Related

» Stroke Prevention

ADHD

Considered a developmental disorder among children, attention deficit hyperactivity disorder (ADHD) is a controversial condition. Whereas medical diagnoses are typically based on symptoms described by a patient, medical history, physical examination by a doctor, and lab tests, ADHD diagnoses in children are based on other people's observations, mostly teachers and, to a lesser degree, parents. There are no medical tests for diagnosis. In some cases, teachers and parents disagree, and a child may never manifest the symptoms when seeing a doctor. An official diagnosis requires that a child have six or more manifestations of inattention, hyperactivity, and impulsivity. Unfortunately, many children are diagnosed as having ADHD when, in fact, they are just more creative or more spirited.

Conventional Treatment

Stimulants, such as Adderall or Ritalin, are the most commonly prescribed medications. They may be prescribed only for the hours a child spends in school, or for use all day, every day. To increase compliance with prescriptions, ADHD medications are available in a variety of forms, including tablets, capsules, liquids, and skin patches. Some are short-acting and others last longer or are time-released. ADHD can be the result of brain injury, which would require different treatment. There is a great deal of disagreement among psychiatrists and psychologists as to the true impact of ADHD on our society. Some are of the opinion that putting these children on powerful drugs will "dumb down" some of our most creative minds, thus denying society some of the most creative ideas. Creative people are generally more restless, especially early in life.

My Recommendations

One of the important observations has been the frequent link between food intolerance and ADHD behaviors. Food intolerance is different from food allergies in that it is much less obvious and can present as behavioral problems that don't have an obvious connection to food. Intolerances of cow's milk, soy products, eggs, chocolate, and peanuts are the more commonly known ones, but a child can be intolerant of a great variety of food products, and sometimes food additives

---

INCIDENCE OF ADHD

The number of diagnosed cases of ADHD have been increasing over the years. According to the Centers for Disease Control and Prevention, these were percentages of children diagnosed with the condition in the United States:

- 2003: 7.8%
- 2007: 9.5%
- 2011: 11%

Compared to girls, boys are more than twice as likely to be diagnosed with ADHD. Overall rates vary substantially by state, from a low of 5.6 percent in Nevada to a high of 18.7 percent in Kentucky. Based on the premise that some children will continue to manifest ADHD as adults, it is estimated that the condition may affect approximately 4 percent of adults in the United States, but this is likely an unrealistically high estimate.

---

or spices. A number of labs offer extensive testing for a large number of foods and spices, such as Alcat (www.alcat.com), Genova Diagnostics (www.gdx.net), and Doctor's Data (www. doctorsdata.com).

Studies have found that these are some of the major substances that trigger ADHD behaviors:

Artificial food coloring: The greater the exposure, the more likely the behavioral effect. Among small children, colored cereals are a major source but artificial colors, often several in combination, are found in many drinks and foods, including candy.

Sugar and starch: These cause the brain to release high concentrations of glutamate, a powerful excitotoxin (see chapter 2) that influences impulsivity, agitation, anxiety, anger and restlessness.

Toxins: Children ages six to fifteen exposed to pyrethroid, a very commonly used insecticide, are twice as likely to develop ADHD as those without exposure. Phthalates, a family of chemicals used in plastics, have also been linked to ADHD, ADD, and learning disorders. Children should not be exposed to pesticides or insecticides and should not eat or drink from plastic containers.

Chronic deficiencies in a number of nutrients are commonly seen in children with ADHD, including zinc, magnesium, iron, iodine, and omega-3 fatty acids, which are found in fish oil.

Natural Supplements
▶ Fish Oil

A number of studies have found a strong link between low omega-3 levels in the blood and brains of children and ADHD or ADD. When omega-3 oils, found in fish, were added to their diets, there was a significant improvement in behavior. Some studies found even better results when omega-3 oils were combined with phosphatidylserine or vitamin D3. Fish oil supplements for children should be high in DHA, one of the two key omega-3 fats (the other is EPA). One good product for children is Carlson for Kids Chewable DHA, which is naturally orange flavored, and for adults, Super DHA Gems, also made by Carlson. Carlson's liquid Fish Oil—either lemon or orange flavored—can also be used. It has high levels of both EPA and DHA components.

➡ **What to do:** Children between the ages of two and six should take 200 mg of DHA a day. From ages seven to fifteen, the recommended dose is 200 mg, twice a day with food. Adults can take 1,000 to 2,000 mg a day as the liquid form with food.

▶ **Phosphatidylserine**

This is a natural lipid, meaning a waxy substance found in all cells and very important in brain cells. It has been found to reduce ADHD symptoms.

➡ **What to do:** For younger children, the usual dose is 50 mg a day, and 100 mg a day after age seven. Adults can take 100 mg, two to three times a day with food.

▶ **Vitamin D3**

Studies have shown that vitamin D3 plays a major role in improving ADHD symptoms, especially when combined with fish oil.

➡ **What to do:** For younger children, the usual dose is 1,000 IU a day, and after age seven through adulthood, 1,000 to 2,000 IU a day.

▶ **Pycnogenol**

An extract from French maritime pine bark, pycnogenol has powerful antioxidant effects, and a number of studies have shown benefits for children with ADHD. Animal studies show that it enhances levels of the body's major internal antioxidant, glutathione, which helps to protect brain cells.

➡ **What to do:** Small children can take 50 mg a day with food, and after age seven through adulthood, 100 mg, one to three times a day with meals.

▶ Multivitamin/Mineral

A well-balanced children's multivitamin/mineral supplement will correct deficiencies in iodine, magnesium, and zinc. Older children, over the age of 12, may need higher doses of magnesium. A slow-release form is best, such as Magnesium w/SRT, made by Jigsaw Health.

➡ **What to do:** Follow multivitamin/mineral label instructions. After age 12, the dose of a slow-release magnesium is 250 mg a day.

▶ Hyperbaric Oxygen Therapy (HBOT)

Private HBOT clinics have reported numerous cases of significant improvement in ADD and ADHD. Both of these disorders are related to excitotoxicity, which HBOT has been shown to reduce.

Alzheimer's, Parkinson's, and ALS

While these are separate diseases, they share the characteristics of deteriorating brain function, a long development period, and no cure by traditional medicine. When researchers examined what increased the risk of these disorders, they found that all had two things in common:

- They increase brain inflammation.

- They trigger excitotoxicity, a very harmful overstimulation of cells in the brain and nervous system.

To describe this newly discovered combination of mechanisms, I coined the term "immunoexcitotoxicity," described in more detail in chapter 2.

Despite their similar underpinnings, each of these conditions has some unique characteristics and symptoms:

TOXINS INCREASE RISK

There are links between diseases that destroy cells in the brain and nervous system and exposure to toxic metals or chemicals. Such links are more common when individuals are continually exposed to these in their jobs or homes. Examples include people who work with agricultural chemicals, suffer electric shocks, experience repeated head or spinal trauma, are in the vicinity of very low-frequency electronic emissions, or are continually exposed to toxic metals, such as aluminum, lead, cadmium, and mercury. All three of these diseases are related to exposure to pesticides, herbicides, and fungicides.

Alzheimer's: Plaques and tangles in the brain and loss of connection between nerve cells are considered the key pathological traits. Memory loss, disorientation, confusion, difficulty with language, and unpredictable behavior are symptoms. The rate of progression can vary considerably.

Parkinson's: Cells in the brain and nervous system, which are used to control movement and coordination, slowly die off. Pathological changes involve many areas of the brain. Symptoms include shaking, also known as tremors, difficulty with balance and walking, rigid or stiff muscles, difficulty swallowing, and infrequent blinking.

ALS: Short for amyotrophic lateral sclerosis, ALS is also known as Lou Gehrig's disease. Cells in the brain and spinal cord, which control muscle movement, progressively die off. Muscles weaken, especially in the arms and legs, and these limbs atrophy, meaning they waste away and become smaller. Speech, breathing, and other functions are also affected, possibly to the point of complete paralysis in later stages.

Conventional Treatment

Different drugs are designed to treat symptoms and, in some individual cases, may slow the progression. The response to these drugs varies among individuals and there are always side effects. Some medications, such as those that replace dopamine, can actually make the disease progress faster.

For Parkinson's, electrical stimulation of the brain, called deep brain stimulation, is sometimes performed and, in rare cases, stem cell implants are used. In the case of ALS, physical therapy, speech therapy, and ventilators to assist with breathing are used to treat symptoms but have no effect on progression or outcome. Newer classes of drugs are being designed and tested for ALS. With all these conditions, good nutrition can improve the quality of life.

👍 My Recommendations

Prevention of these neurodegenerative diseases should begin early in life, with breast feeding and avoiding excess vaccinations during childhood, which can set the stage for later-life neurodegeneration. At all ages, avoid exposure to pesticides, herbicides, and fungicides, in the home, garden, and workplace. Living near a farm or golf course can increase your risk.

Other common toxins that should be avoided include:

- Dental amalgam fillings, which contain mercury

- Dental products with fluoride, such as toothpaste, mouthwash, and fluoride treatments at the dentist

- Drinking water with fluoride

- Mercury in fish and polluted environments

- Aluminum, which may be added to foods and medications and is in aluminum foil, cans, aluminum cookware, many vaccines, and municipal drinking water

A healthy diet can go a long way in preventing these diseases. This means avoiding sugar and high-starch foods, such as white rice and most grains, especially white breads. Inflammatory omega-6 fats, such as corn, safflower, sunflower, peanut, soybean, and canola oils, should be replaced with coconut oil and extra virgin olive oil, and processed foods should be avoided, as they almost always contain the inflammatory oils. In addition, it's vital to eat at least 10 servings of nutrient-dense vegetables daily. This is more realistic if you make the vegetable drink I suggest in chapter 3, and drink 12 ounces of the mixture, twice a day.

Energy depletion is one of the major defects in many neurodegenerative diseases, especially Alzheimer's and Parkinson's. Extra virgin coconut oil contains a particularly beneficial type of oil, called medium chain triglyceride, or MCT for short, which maximizes energy production in the brain and protects against excitotoxicity.

Regular mental exercise is also important, such as playing brain games, reading, memorizing passages and lists, or learning a new language or how to play a musical instrument. Relaxation and stress reduction are also vital, as chronic stress has been shown to increase brain inflammation. Stress reducers include getting a good night's sleep, prayer, and daily moderate exercise. Exercise increases production of brain-derived neurotropic factor, BDNF for short, a substance that enables the brain to repair itself.

Natural Supplements

There are a number of useful compounds to protect against and improve the quality of life where Alzheimer's, ALS, or Parkinson's has developed. I've included the most important ones below.

▶ Curcumin

An extract from the curry spice turmeric, curcumin is therapeutic because it is well established as a powerful anti-inflammatory. Most important, it can calm specific types of immune cells in the brain, called microglia and macrophages, which are central to neurodegeneration. It also raises brain levels of a neurotransmitter called acetylcholine, which improves memory and calms brain inflammation. And, curcumin reduces aluminum toxicity. For best absorption, use CurcumaSorb, made by Pure Encapsulations, which contains 250 mg per capsule.

➡ **What to do:** Take one capsule (250 mg) of CurcumaSorb, three times a day with meals. Because it has a high degree of safety, even in very large doses, you can increase the dose to 500 mg, three times a day with meals. If you use a different product, for best absorption, I recommend opening capsules and mixing the contents with a teaspoon of coconut oil or extra virgin olive oil, taking the mixture, and then drinking some water. This is messy but important, as dry, powdered curcumin is typically not well absorbed.

▶ **Luteolin**

This is a flavonoid found in several plants, such as celery and artichoke. A number of studies have shown that it powerfully reduces brain inflammation by quieting key immune cells, the microglia and macrophages, and immunoexcitotoxicity.

➡ **What to do:** Take 100 mg, three times a day with meals. After one week, the dose can be increased to 300 mg, three times a day with meals.

▶ **Apigenin**

Another flavonoid, apigenin is found in plants such as celery, parsley, and ginkgo biloba. Like luteolin, it reduces brain inflammation and immunoexcitotoxicity. However, since every herbal extract works slightly different, both luteolin and apigenin are beneficial.

➡ **What to do:** Take 50 mg, three times a day with meals. After one week, the dose can be increased to 150 mg, three times a day.

▶ **Magnesium**

Magnesium reduces excitotoxicity and brain inflammation, improves blood flow to the brain, and raises levels of our chief internal antioxidant, glutathione, in brain cells. For best absorption, use a slow-release version of magnesium malate, such as Magnesium w/SRT, made by Jigsaw Health. Two caplets contain 250 mg.

➧ **What to do:** Take two caplets (250 mg), twice a day with meals.

▶ Fish Oil

Omega-3 oil, found in fish, is essential to maintain the fluid-like properties of brain cell connections and membranes. Omgea-3 oils have an EPA component and a DHA component. The vast majority of the brain contains DHA, which can be taken as a fish oil that is high in DHA. One good product for children is Carlson for Kids Chewable DHA, which is naturally orange flavored, and for adults, Super DHA Gems, or a liquid form, Carlson's Fish Oil, both of which are made by Carlson.

➧ **What to do:** Brain health begins in the womb. Pregnant women should take no more than 200 mg a day of DHA. After delivery and during breast feeding, the mother can take 1, 000 mg a day. Children between the ages of two and six should take 200 mg of DHA a day. From age seven to age fifteen, the dose is 200 mg, twice a day with food. Adults and older teenagers can take 1,000 to 2,000 mg a day with food.

▶ Acetyl-L Carnitine and Vinpocetine

A specific form of carnitine, acetyl-L-carnitine is a natural compound that has been shown to enhance brain function. It improves the connections between brain cells, reduces inflammation and excitotoxicity, and improves brain energy production. Vinpocetine is extracted from the periwinkle plant. It raises brain dopamine levels, improves blood flow in the brain, is a powerful anti-inflammatory, and has great potential to reduce neurodegeneration in Alzheimer's and Parkinson's. A specific combination of these, Cresceo-ALC, made by Medix Select, contains 1,500 mg of acetyl-L-carnitine and 30 mg of vinpocetine in two capsules.

➡ **What to do:** Take one Cresceo-ALC capsule, twice a day with meals. The maximum dose is one capsule, three times a day with meals.

▶ R-Lipoic Acid

Naturally found in all cells, this is a very powerful and versatile antioxidant. It reduces excitotoxicity and improves energy production in brain cells. Studies have shown that it offers benefit in treating ALS and other neurodegenerative diseases.

➡ **What to do:** The starting dose is 100 mg, three times a day with meals. The dosage can be increased to 300 to 600 mg, three times a day with meals, which is especially helpful for diabetics.

▶ Pyruvate

Pyruvate is a breakdown product of glucose that improves levels of energy in the brain. This helps to counteract one of the key defects in many neurodegenerative diseases, where the energy-producing components of cells, called mitochondria, are impaired. One of the best sources of pyruvate I have found is Triple Pyruvate Electrolyte Complex, made by Swanson Health Products. Each capsule contains 775 mg of the pyruvate complex.

➡ **What to do:** Take two to three capsules, three times a day with meals.

▶ Resveratrol

Resveratrol is a flavonoid found in high concentrations in grape skins. It has been shown to extend lifespan in animals, and it reduces excitotoxicity and inflammation. Resveratrol also improves insulin function, which is a major player in Alzheimer's disease.

➡ **What to take:** The optimal dose is 200 to 250 mg a day, with food. Higher doses can have negative effects on cellular energy production.

▶ Niacinamide (vitamin B3)

It plays a major role in energy production by all cells, including brain cells. When combined with resveratrol, we see synergistic benefits of enhanced energy production and brain protection.

➡ **What to do:** The usual dose is 500 mg, two to three times a day with meals.

▶ Multivitamin/Mineral

People at risk of neurodegenerative disorders need adequate intake of all of the major vitamins and minerals. Iron should not be in your supplement, as in most cases of neurodegenerative diseases, we see excess iron in the brain and spinal cord. A good product should include all of the B vitamins in an absorbable form, such as the "5-methyltetrahydrofolate" form of folic acid, multiple forms of natural vitamin E, some vitamin C, and the trace minerals.

➡ **What to do:** Follow directions for the product you choose.

▶ Methylcobalamin (vitamin B12)

This is the most absorbable and beneficial form of vitamin B12, which is essential for energy production in the brain but often in short supply among older people. I prefer a sublingual form, which dissolves under the tongue.

➡ **What to do:** Take 10,000 mcg a day of a sublingual form.

▶ Hyperbaric Oxygen Therapy (HBOT)

There have been no well-controlled human studies of HBOT in the treatment of these neurodegenerative diseases, but case studies have shown that some patients improve, a few rather dramatically. Inflammation is central to all these disorders and the ability of HBOT to reduce inflammation holds much promise for improving symptoms and slowing the progression of these debilitating conditions. Some animal studies of neurodegenerative diseases have shown improvement with HBOT.

Lack of oxygen is universal in these disorders and HBOT can raise oxygen levels in deep brain tissue that cannot be reached by other means.

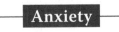

Anxiety

Faced with an unexpected situation, at work or in one's personal life, it isn't uncommon to feel a little anxious. In fact, anxiety is a normal reaction, especially when dealing with changing circumstances or unfamiliar challenges. For example, people often feel worried or anxious when meeting new people, taking a test, starting a new job, or making an important decision. However, if worry or anxiety becomes a constant problem, it requires attention.

Anxiety may manifest as a sense of uneasiness or worry, irritability, fatigue, muscle tension, and even muscle aches or headaches. Severe anxiety may lead to panic attacks, with physical symptoms such as sweating, dizziness, and heart palpitations, or unprovoked but constant worry. There are no lab tests to diagnose anxiety as a disorder. Physical or mental stress in life is one trigger, and more recent evidence shows that chronic inflammation, as a result of a poor diet and exposure to toxins, is another all too common one.

> **SIDE EFFECTS OF DRUGS**
>
> Anxiety may be a side effect of antidepressants, which can also cause memory loss, fatigue, nausea, or dizziness. For antianxiety drugs, side effects may include:
>
> - Stomach upset
> - Confusion
> - Disorientation
> - Blurred vision
> - Slurred speech
> - Slowed mental and physical reaction

Conventional Treatment

Tranquilizers can lead to a dependence as well as many serious side effects. A significant number of people fail to respond to pharmaceutical treatments, even when multiple drugs are used. All too often, physicians rely heavily on such medications and don't fully educate patients about common side effects. Or, they don't disclose that when the drugs are stopped, the original condition is likely to rebound in a more intense way. In many cases, anxiety is a symptom of an underlying physical condition, but drugs to treat the symptom are prescribed in place of a thorough evaluation and correct diagnosis.

👍 My Recommendations

Newer research is finding that diet plays a significant role in our mental health. Some foods and food additives increase brain inflammation. These include inflammatory omega-6 vegetable oils, such as corn, soy, safflower, sunflower, and peanut oils, sugar, and high protein diets, and they can worsen depression and anxiety. On an immediate basis, sugar or starchy foods may seem to bring relief from anxiety but, over the long run, will perpetuate difficulties.

In people who suffer from very severe drops in blood sugar, a condition called reactive hypoglycemia, sugar can cause severe attacks of anxiety and even panic attacks. When the brain's energy supply begins to fail, as happens with low blood sugar, special brain cells, called microglia and astrocytes, release high levels of inflammatory chemicals and glutamate. For an explanation of glutamate and excitotoxicity, see chapter 2.

A healthy diet, which is also covered in chapter 1, contains these: anti-inflammatory omega-3 oils, especially the DHA component of fish oil; at least 10 servings of vegetables; a mixture of complex carbohydrates, such as beans, whole grain organic rice, and blueberries; and purified water. Vegetables in the drink I describe in chapter 3 are easier to consume in quantity, and nutrients are more effectively absorbed, than by eating platefuls of whole raw vegetables. Soy products should be avoided, as they are a major source of glutamate, as well as high levels of fluoride, which is toxic.

This type of diet can reduce brain inflammation and excitotoxicity. Once it becomes routine, attacks of anxiety will be less likely. Regular exercise also counteracts anxiety, as it raises levels of endorphins, natural feel-good chemicals. Stress is a major contributor to anxiety and can be reduced by regular exercise, learning to compartmentalize your life, becoming involved in community or religious activities, developing social bonds, and living each day to its fullest.

Natural Supplements

▶ Gastrodin

Studies of gastrodin, an extract from a Chinese herb called Gastrodia elata, show that it may relieve anxiety by reducing brain inflammation and excitotoxicity. And, it protects brain stem cells, which reverses shrinkage of the hippocampal area of the brain and protects memory.

> ➡ **What to do:** Take 300 mg, once a day for a week, and then take the same amount twice a day. For severe anxiety, increase the dose to two 300 mg capsules, twice a day. Always take it with food.

▶ Fish Oil

Omega-3 oil, found in fish, is essential for maintaining the fluid-like properties of brain cell connections and membranes. Omega-3 oils contain two key components: EPA and DHA. The majority of the brain contains mostly DHA, which is essential for brain development in the womb and during childhood and for brain protection throughout life.

> ➡ **What to do:** A liquid Norwegian Fish Oil with either a lemon or orange natural flavor, made by Carlson, is a pure product with high concentrations of DHA. Take two

teaspoons, twice a day. For severe anxiety, increase the dose to a tablespoon, twice a day.

▶ Hesperidin Methyl Chalcone

This is a specific form of hesperidin, a compound commonly found in oranges. Several studies have shown that it not only acts as an antianxiety compound, but also protects the brain.

➡ **What to do:** Take 500 mg, three times a day with meals.

▶ Magnesium

Magnesium reduces excitotoxicity and brain inflammation, improves blood flow to the brain, and raises levels of our internal antioxidant glutathione, which protects brain cells. For best absorption, take a slow-release form of magnesium malate, such as Magnesium w/SRT, made by Jigsaw Health, which provides 500 mg of magnesium in two caplets.

➡ **What to do:** Take two caplets, twice a day with meals.

▶ Tyrosine

A number of studies have shown that tyrosine, an amino acid, can reduce anxiety and stress and elevate mood.

➡ **What to do:** Take 500 mg, three times a day, 45 minutes before each meal.

▶ Hyperbaric Oxygen Therapy (HBOT)

There are a great many triggers for anxiety, such as inflammation, a poor diet, certain toxic metal exposures, and diseases that cause hypoxia, meaning low oxygen levels in the body. In all of these conditions, the brain releases too much glutamate, an excitotoxin that triggers anxiety. Reducing excitotoxicity and inflammation calms the anxiety and depression. HBOT effectively addresses all of these problems.

Brain Aging

As we live longer, there are changes in the entire human body, including the brain and nervous system. There is evidence that with age, some brain regions shrink and other changes occur in neurons that make up the nervous system. Blood flow to the brain may be reduced because blood vessels narrow or become less flexible. However, such changes do not necessarily have an effect on an individual's mental abilities and there is no innate reason why any dementia or other neurodegenerative condition should develop. In fact, language abilities may improve as people live longer. There is an old observation that the aged brain works slower than the younger brain, but its complexity is much greater, thus allowing deeper and more complex thinking—something we call cognitive ability.

No one has defined "normal" brain aging, but being able to maintain one's independence is certainly critical. Of course, one would like to have a mind and memory that works as well as when we were in college, but only the rare individual attains that goal. Evidence shows that the cognitive state of an older individual is a result of a great number of factors. Genetics play a role, but lifestyle influences which genes are turned on or off—an ongoing process of gene regulation called epigenetics.

Many elements play important roles, including education,

> **HEALTHY BRAIN AGING**
>
> Overall good health contributes to healthy brain aging. This includes doing the things that reduce the risk of diabetes and promote a healthy heart, such as controlling blood pressure and inflammation and:
>
> - Maintaining a healthy weight
> - Being physically active in the course of each day
> - Getting additional regular exercise through regular activity or formal fitness programs
> - Eating a healthy diet with plenty of vegetables and fruits
> - Staying engaged intellectually, through work and charitable activities, and by learning new skills
> - Being involved in community activities
> - Maintaining close ties with family and friends

diet, fitness level, occupation, recreational activities, other life experiences, and stress, especially when chronic or intense. Brain aging is intensified by exposure to environmental toxins, including mercury, lead, cadmium, tin, manganese, industrial chemicals, and agricultural chemicals such as pesticides, herbicides, and fungicides.

All the factors associated with pathological brain aging have this in common: they all cause brain inflammation that sets off destructive processes. These first destroy the synapses and dendrites, critical links between neurons, and over time the neurons can die off, at which point the brain shrinks appreciably. However, much of this can be reversed, especially in the early stages.

Conventional Treatment

The natural aging process is not a disease and does not have a medical treatment. However, where there is a medical or dental condition which can be effectively treated, such as a known viral or bacterial infection, receiving the appropriate treatment will improve the overall health of the body. This will increase well-being and the ability to stay mentally engaged and both physically and mentally active. And these actions will, in turn, help maintain a healthy brain and nervous system.

Most doctors will instruct their elderly patients to avoid stress, eat healthy, exercise regularly, and get plenty of rest. For many people, these things are not easily done and require a little more in the way of specific instructions.

My Recommendations

Diet is critical for brain health. The structure of the human body, including the brain, is constantly being replaced. As an example, the brain you have now is not the one you had 10 years ago. To continually rebuild healthy structure and function properly, the human body requires all the necessary building blocks—nutrients. Only then can all the cells, brain connections, receptors, blood vessels, and other tissues heal from routine damage, deal with life's challenges, and remain in good shape.

The overall diet that provides good building blocks is described in the first few chapters of this book but for healthy brain aging, these are some of the most important points:

Eat vegetables and berries. Vegetables contain thousands of compounds that rebuild damaged cells and brain connections and defend against destructive inflammation. For example, spinach, broccoli, Brussels sprouts, and other cruciferous vegetables contain flavonoids and other powerful brain-protective chemicals. Blueberries slow brain aging and reverse a good deal of age-related damage, and blackberries, raspberries, and strawberries are also very beneficial. Cacao (dark chocolate), if organically grown, supplies a number of important brain-protecting molecules. I recommend blenderizing vegetables, as described in the "Drink Your Veggies" chapter.

Get the right fats. Avoid inflammatory oils that are commonly used, especially for deep frying, but are powerful triggers of brain inflammation. These include corn, peanut, soybean, safflower, and sunflower oils. They easily enter the brain and do a great deal of damage. Trans fats, in partially hydrogenated oils, interfere with brain cell communication and cause additional brain inflammation. In contrast, the anti-inflammatory omega-3 oils found in fish, especially DHA, play a critical role in brain health. DHA is a major building block of neurons, the cells that make up the brain and nervous system.

Get enough vitamin D3. Lack of vitamin D3 speeds aging of the brain, and even people in sunny climates are often deficient. Get vitamin D3 checked with a blood test from your doctor, and take the amount needed to get and maintain your vitamin D blood levels between 65 and 100 ng/ml.

Avoid fluoride. A highly toxic metal, fluoride accumulates in certain areas of the brain (the pineal gland and hippocampus) and has been shown to significantly lower IQ and interfere with memory and complex brain functions. Studies have shown that even concentrations of 0.5 parts per million (ppm) can damage cells and microvessels in the brain. Yet, 60 percent of our public drinking water is fluorinated at higher levels of 1 to 1.3 ppm.

Drink beneficial beverages. Black tea has very high levels of fluoride but white and green teas have very low levels. In addition, white and green teas are high in catechins, compounds that protect the brain. Coffee also contains a number of antioxidants that can protect the brain. Drink these hot or iced, especially white tea, the richest in compounds that benefit the brain.

Drink fluoride-free water. To avoid fluoride, drink filtered or distilled water. If you drink distilled water, add about 150 mg of magnesium citrate or malate powder to each gallon, to replace minerals lost during distillation. Magnesium powder, made by Pure Encapsulations, is a good product.

Limit sugar. Sugar is the great brain destroyer. Other starchy carbohydrates, such as white breads, white rice, and pasta are also wrecking our brains. Both of these types of foods are far too abundant in typical American diets. My favorite sugar replacement is a product called Just Like Sugar®.

Beware of gluten. For some people, gluten in grain can rob brain function and even lead to serious neurological disorders, such as seizures and possibly schizophrenia. Reaction to gluten varies among individuals. Some people can tolerate certain amounts while others can tolerate none, so it's important to know what is right for you (for more details, see the section "Celiac Disease and Gluten" in chapter 9). Many gluten free products are made with rice or potato flour, which can trigger intense hypoglycemia in some people.

Exercise. Often underrated, exercise is essential for a healthy brain. It triggers release of endorphins, chemicals that reduce pain, boost mood, and stimulate production of special compounds that repair and build new brain structures, such as dendrites and synapses. Brisk walking is good, but resistance exercises working all the major muscles is equally, if not more, important. Do these for 30 minutes to an hour, five days a week.

Socialize and single-task. Having in-person conversations with friends and family has been shown to overcome a number of serious brain-damaging events. It is far superior to electronic and even phone communication. In contrast, multitasking destroys our ability to focus attention and negatively affects learning and deeper thinking.

Maintain healthy digestion. Gut inflammation, such as that caused by food allergies or intolerance, can cause chronic brain inflammation and eventual neurodegeneration, leading to anxiety, depression, and cognitive impairment. Inflammation can also be generated by an imbalance of bacteria in the digestive tract. A variety of tests, such as those offered by Doctor's Data (www.doctorsdata.com) and Alcat (www.alcat.com), which must be ordered and evaluated by a health professional, can identify problems so that these can be corrected. If you have certain digestive symptoms, see the related section in chapter 9, "Digestion," and for more about gut inflammation, see the section on "Crohn's and Other Inflammatory Bowel Diseases."

Natural Supplements

▶ Curcumin

Curcumin is a flavonoid found in higher concentrations in the curry spice turmeric. Many studies have found it to be a very powerful compound for protecting the brain against aging, Alzheimer's, and other neurodegenerative diseases. It is a very powerful antioxidant, improves blood flow, and dissolves amyloid plaque related to Alzheimer's. Studies using massive doses found it to have a very high margin of safety. When dissolved in an oil, such as coconut or extra virgin olive oil, it is well absorbed and enters the brain very easily from the blood.

➡ **What to do:** Take 250 to 500 mg, three times a day, with meals. Use a highly absorbable form such as CurcumaSorb, made by Pure Encapsulations. Or, mix the powder contents of a capsule with a tablespoon of coconut or extra virgin olive oil. This can be messy.

▶ Quercetin

This is a flavonoid found in plants, such as tea, onions, parsley, and apples. It has powerful antioxidant and anti-inflammatory effects and is even more effective when taken with curcumin.

➡ **What to do:** Take 250 to 500 mg, three times a day, of a form that is well absorbed, such as Quercenase, made by Thorne Research.

▶ Resveratrol

This is a flavonoid that is concentrated in the skins of grapes and is found in varying quantities in red wine. Resveratrol protects the brain, stimulates natural repair mechanisms, and is a powerful antioxidant. It also improves metabolism of blood sugar in the brain, which is essential for its healthy function. High doses should be taken with niacinamide, a B vitamin, as high resveratrol doses can lead to cellular energy depletion.

➡ **What to do:** Take between 200 and 250 mg a day with food. If you take more than 300 mg daily, also take 500 mg of niacinamide daily.

▶ Gastrodin

An active component of the Chinese tall gastrodia tuber, Gastrodin has been used to treat a number of neurological problems, including dizziness. It has powerful neuroprotective effects, enhances memory, improves natural repair mechanisms, and stimulates the brain to release higher levels of GABA, a protective neurotransmitter. It improves blood supply to the brain, has a calming effect, relieves pain, suppresses excitotoxicity, inhibits seizures, and neutralizes free radicals.

➤ **What to do:** Take one capsule (300 mg), twice a day, with or without food. Gastrodin can be found in Brain Shield Gastrodin, made by Life Extension. The dose can be increased to no more than two capsules, two to three times a day, as needed.

▶ Bacopa Monnieri (Brahmi)

A plant extract from India, Bacopa monnieri is nicknamed "brahmi." Studies have found that it improves memory and concentration, inhibits age-related brain inflammation, enhances brain flexibility, and inhibits seizures. It is safe when taken in recommended doses, but higher doses have been associated with a slow heart rate and could possibly increase fluid secretion in the intestines and lungs. It should not be used during pregnancy or breast feeding.

➤ **What to do:** Follow product directions.

▶ Vinpocetine

Derived from the periwinkle plant, Vinpocetine increases blood flow in the brain and is a powerful anti-inflammatory compound. It protects brain cells, reduces stroke damage, can improve some hearing disorders, reduces tinnitus, and has anti-seizure properties.

➤ **What to do:** Take 10 to 20 mg, three times a day, with meals.

▶ DHA

Short for docosahexaenoic acid, DHA is a component of omega-3 oils found in fish. It is one of the most abundant fats in the brain and is a building block of neuron membranes and junctions between nerve cells, called synapses. Studies show that DHA protects against degeneration associated with repetitive head injuries. It plays a major role in brain development, inhibits excitotoxicity, and reduces brain inflammation. The brain contains very little EPA, the other key component of fish oil. DHA is also found in certain types of algae.

➭ **What to do:** Take 1,000 to 2,000 mg a day of DHA, from fish oil or algae.

▶ Mixed Tocopherols and Tocotrienols

In nature, vitamin E is a family of nutrients composed of four compounds called tocopherols and four compounds called tocotrienols. Together, they have strong antioxidant and anti-inflammatory effects, and protect the brain and nervous system.

➭ **What to do:** Take 400 IU of mixed tocopherols and 50 mg of mixed tocotrienols, twice a day with meals.

▶ Buffered Vitamin C

Although vitamin C is known to be an antioxidant, it does much more. It regulates neurotransmitters, reduces inflammation, enhances immunity, stimulates cellular energy production, and has anticancer, antiviral, and antibacterial effects. Lypo-Spheric Vitamin C, made by LivOn Labs, is a highly absorbable, buffered form that is non-acidic and easy on the stomach. It comes in packets of gel that can be mixed with water or other liquids. When taken with food, vitamin C increases absorption of iron and can lead to iron overload, which is harmful to the brain. High doses of ordinary vitamin C supplements, which are usually acidic, can cause digestive upset.

➭ **What to do:** Take 1 packet (1,000 mg) of Lypo-Spheric Vitamin C, three times a day between meals.

▶ B Vitamins

The B vitamins are essential for our bodies to convert food into energy. This is especially important for healthy aging of the brain, which uses a tremendous amount of energy to perform its normal around-the-clock functions. In addition, the brain has special receptors for most of the B vitamins, especially for vitamins

B2 (riboflavin), thiamine, and B6 (pyridoxine). B6 also plays a vital part in neurotransmitter function and calming the central nervous system by inhibiting excessive glutamate elevations in the brain and blood (explained in the "Excitotoxins" chapter).

All the B vitamins work together and help to protect the brain. They are best taken in a B-complex supplement that is bioavailable, meaning easily absorbed and utilized by the human body. Regular B vitamin supplements need to be converted into their active form in the digestive system and liver, but if these are not functioning optimally, the vitamins cannot be efficiently utilized and will not deliver benefits. The absorbable forms have specific names, such as riboflavin 5'-phosphate for vitamin B2 and pyridoxal 5-phosphate for vitamin B6. The Activated B-Complex High Bioavailability Formula, made by Swanson, contains a good combination of B vitamins in absorbable forms.

➡ **What to do:** Take one capsule a day of the Swanson Activated B-Complex High Bioavailability Formula, with or without food.

▶ Selenium (Selenomethionine)

As with B vitamins, selenium needs to be taken in an absorbable form, called selenomethionine. This essential trace mineral helps our bodies produce a very important internal antioxidant found in all our cells, called glutathione peroxidase, and is vital for proper detoxification. Both of these functions protect the brain and help it to function well through a long life. Selenium also has anticancer effects.

➡ **What to do:** Take 100 mcg a day.

▶ Magnesium

The fourth most abundant mineral in the body, magnesium has powerful anti-inflammatory effects, plays a critical role in metabolism and immunity, improves blood flow, and has antioxidant properties. In addition, it blocks excitotoxic reactions, which would otherwise damage the brain and central nervous system. Many people are deficient in magnesium and will require a higher intake of the mineral. Some lower-cost forms, such as magnesium oxide or chloride, are generally poorly absorbed and can cause severe diarrhea. In contrast, magnesium citrate, malate, or threonate are well absorbed, much less likely to cause diarrhea or other digestive upset, and enhance healthy energy production that is vital for proper brain function. The threonate form is especially well absorbed in the brain. In animal studies, it has reversed Alzheimer's disease, but this has not been tested in human cases.

> ➡ **What to do:** I prefer a slow-release form of magnesium malate called Magnesium w/SRT, made by Jigsaw Health. Take two caplets, two or three times a day, with meals. Or, take a magnesium L-threonate supplement with an ingredient called Magtein listed in the Supplement Facts section of the product label. Three capsules make up one daily dose of 2,000 mg. A number of companies make products with this dose. I prefer to take both forms.

▶ Zinc

The brain normally contains high concentrations of zinc, especially in the hippocampus and cortex, but most elderly are quite deficient in the mineral. Zinc inhibits excitotoxicity and has anti-inflammatory properties. However, excess zinc in the brain is suspected to cause damage to synapses.

> ➡ **What to do:** The maintenance dose of zinc is 15 mg a day but severe deficiencies require higher amounts, based on blood tests of zinc levels.

▶ Hyperbaric Oxygen Therapy (HBOT)

Hyperbaric oxygen treatment, with 100 percent oxygen at increased atmospheric pressures, holds much promise in reversing mild cognitive impairment associated not only with aging, but also with strokes, head injuries, and other neurological problems.

Several studies, with humans and animals, have demonstrated some dramatic benefits. HBOT has been shown to reduce brain inflammation, stimulate production of brain stem cells, increase antioxidant defenses, and speed the reversal of atherosclerosis. In people with long-term neuroborreliosis, a disorder of the central nervous system resulting from Lyme disease, HBOT has produced dramatic improvement in short-term memory. All these improvements persist long after HBOT treatments, and if they begin to reverse, one can repeat the treatments.

Depression

It isn't uncommon to feel a little blue from time to time, when life events are disappointing or too challenging, but when the feeling persists, it can become a problem. Depression may manifest as a sad or hopeless feeling, low energy, and a loss of interest in activities that are usually enjoyable. In major depression, one cannot delineate a definite cause—it just seems to come out of the blue. Unlike occasional depression, it can be progressive and overwhelming and can lead to major disability.

Our understanding of major depression has changed considerably. Compelling evidence suggests that chronic inflammation and excitotoxicity, which together make up immunoexcitotoxicity (explained in chapter 2), play a major role. Chronic inflammatory disorders, such as autoimmune diseases, arthritis, latent infections, and aging itself, can all result in depression. In many cases, the depression appears before the disease is clinically evident, as the inflammation can be quite subtle for many years.

This new hypothesis explains the common association between major depression, memory loss, and atrophy of part of the brain. It also explains why there is a long delay between taking an antidepressant and its beneficial effects. The drugs that work have anti-inflammatory effects, but it takes several weeks before those effects fully manifest.

⌒ Conventional Treatment

Antidepressants are proving not to be as effective as was once believed, especially for major depression. A significant number of people fail to respond to pharmaceutical treatments, even when multiple drugs are used. Physicians rely heavily on such medications and all too often don't fully educate patients about common side effects. Or, they don't disclose that when the drugs are stopped, the original condition is likely to rebound in a more intense way. In many cases, depression is a symptom of an underlying physical condition, but drugs to treat the symptom are prescribed in place of a thorough evaluation and correct diagnosis.

👍 My Recommendations

Newer research is finding that diet plays a significant role in our mental health. Some foods and food additives increase brain inflammation. These include inflammatory omega-6 vegetable oils, such as corn, soy, safflower, sunflower, and peanut oils, sugar, and high protein diets, and they can worsen depression. On an immediate basis, sugar can boost mood and make us feel "happy," but over the long run it will cause a condition of progressive depression.

Eating a high-sugar, high-starch diet can eventually lead to very severe drops in blood sugar. And then, special brain cells, called microglia and astrocytes, release high

---

SIDE EFFECTS OF DRUGS

Depression may be a side effect of antianxiety medications. Side effects of antidepressants include:

- Memory loss
- Fatigue
- Nausea
- Dizziness
- Weight gain
- Sexual problems
- Insomnia
- Tremors
- Sweating
- Constipation
- Diarrhea
- Dry mouth
- Headaches

levels of inflammatory chemicals and glutamate. For an explanation of glutamate and excitotoxicity, see chapter 2.

A healthy diet, which is also covered in chapter 1, contains these: anti-inflammatory omega-3 oils, especially the DHA component of fish oil; at least 10 servings of vegetables; a mixture of complex carbohydrates, such as beans, whole grain organic rice, and blueberries; and purified water. Vegetables in the drink I describe in chapter 3 are easier to consume in quantity, and nutrients are more effectively absorbed, than by eating platefuls of whole raw vegetables. Soy products should be avoided, as they are a major source of glutamate, as well as high levels of fluoride, which is toxic. This type of diet can reduce brain inflammation and excitotoxicity. Once it becomes routine, depression will subside.

Regular exercise also counteracts depression, as it raises levels of endorphins, natural feel-good chemicals that elevate mood. Even more important, exercise increases brain levels of a brain-cell growth factor that has been shown to relieve depression and protect against depression-induced brain shrinkage.

Stress is a major contributor to depression, as it inflames the brain. Stress-relieving techniques, such as taking time off from work, regular exercise, learning to compartmentalize your life, becoming involved in community or religious activities, developing social bonds, and living each day to its fullest, will go a long way in reducing depression.

Natural Supplements

▶ Gastrodin

Studies of gastrodin, an extract from a Chinese herb called Gastrodia elata, show that it may relieve depression by reducing brain inflammation and excitotoxicity. And, it protects brain stem cells, which reverses shrinkage of the hippocampal area of the brain and protects memory.

> ➡ **What to do:** Take 300 mg, once a day for a week, and then take the same amount twice a day. For severe depression,

increase the dose to two 300 mg capsules, twice a day. Always take it with food.

▶ Fish Oil

Omega-3 oil, found in fish, is essential for maintaining the fluid-like properties of brain cell connections and membranes. Omega-3 oils contain two key components: EPA and DHA. The majority of the brain contains mostly DHA, which is essential for brain development in the womb and during childhood, and for brain protection throughout life.

➡ **What to do:** A liquid Norwegian Fish Oil with either a lemon or orange natural flavor, made by Carlson, is a pure product with high concentrations of DHA. Take two teaspoons, twice a day. For severe depression, increase the dose to a tablespoon, twice a day.

▶ Magnesium

Magnesium reduces excitotoxicity and brain inflammation, improves blood flow to the brain, and raises levels of our chief internal antioxidant, glutathione, which protects brain cells. For best absorption, take a slow-release form of magnesium malate, such as Magnesium w/SRT, made by Jigsaw Health, which provides 500 mg of magnesium in two caplets.

➡ **What to do:** Take two caplets, twice a day with meals.

▶ Tyrosine

A number of studies have shown that tyrosine, an amino acid, can reduce stress and elevate mood.

➡ **What to do:** Take 500 mg, three times a day, 45 minutes before each meal.

▶ Hyperbaric Oxygen Therapy (HBOT)

Depression and anxiety frequently go together and are both caused by inflammation and excitotoxicity within special areas of the brain. HBOT reduces brain inflammation and excitotoxicity. HBOT also improves energy, and this also relieves depression.

Memory Loss, Age-Related

Some brain cells are lost with age, but significant memory loss is not an inevitable consequence of aging. At any time of life, it isn't uncommon to be temporarily forgetful as a result of insufficient sleep, jet lag, or exceptionally stressful or challenging situations, but serious, persistent memory lapses indicate an underlying condition—not necessarily any type of dementia. At the same time, some people maintain exceptional abilities to remember throughout a long life.

Chronic inflammation is a major contributing factor in what is technically called "minimal cognitive impairment" (MCI), also known as "senior moments." In such situations, there is a link between low-grade, chronic brain inflammation and excitotoxicity, described in more detail in chapter 2. A growing number of triggers for such inflammation occur throughout life, including chronic infections, repeated injury, recurrent mini-strokes, stress, autoimmune diseases, excessive vaccination, and exposure to a number of toxic substances. Older people frequently take a number of prescription drugs, many of which impair brain function.

Conventional Treatment

There is no drug or other medical treatment to prevent memory loss or improve memory. If forgetfulness

COMMON DRUGS THAT CAUSE MEMORY LOSS

Many drugs may cause memory loss as a side effect. Common ones include those prescribed for:

- Allergies (antihistamines)
- Anxiety
- Cholesterol lowering (statins)
- Depression
- High blood pressure
- Incontinence
- Insomnia
- Pain (narcotics)
- Parkinson's
- Seizures

becomes a problem, it should be treated as a symptom, rather than a disease, and a competent doctor should evaluate the individual's overall health, including possible prescription drugs that could be causing the problem. Medical situations that may affect memory include brain injuries and disorders, imbalances of sex or thyroid hormones, stroke, severe illness, surgery, and cancer treatment.

👍 My Recommendations

There are two basic principles of protection—avoid the things that damage the brain and take more of the things that protect the brain. For example, these are things to avoid: toxic metals such as mercury, aluminum, cadmium, lead, and excess manganese; pesticides, herbicides, and fungicides; toxic industrial chemicals; black and other mold toxins; and toxins in food. Dietary toxic substances include inflammatory omega-6 oils (corn, safflower, sunflower, peanut, and soybean oils), excess sugar, excess red meats, foods and additives high in glutamate (listed in chapter 2), and fluoridated drinking water.

Regular, moderate exercise is important—at least 30 minutes a day. Prayer should be a regular part of your life. Establishing good friendships is very important and this includes maintaining close family ties. Reading, learning new things, such as a new language or playing a musical instrument, and just exploring the world around you can bring great stress relief. One should develop a proper perspective in regard to time to relax and time to work. It is important not to let material goals dominate your life.

Vegetables and fruits are among the most powerful brain-protecting foods, especially high-nutrient ones. Among vegetables, these include kale, broccoli, Brussels sprouts, cabbage, cauliflower, garlic, onions, and spinach, and among fruits: strawberries, blueberries, blackberries, raspberries, and acai berries. Eat organically grown ones, as they are far superior to conventionally grown varieties. I recommend making a vegetable drink, per my recipe in chapter 3, and drinking 12 ounces of the mixture, twice a day.

🐰 Natural Supplements

▶ Fish Oil

In fish oil, which contains beneficial omega-3 fats, there are two major components, EPA and DHA. Of these, DHA is most concentrated in the brain and is essential for maintaining fluidity, flexibility, and integrity of brain cell connections and membranes. DHA (and EPA) must be obtained from diet, since our bodies do not make these. Not all fish oil supplements contain high doses of DHA. One that does, and I recommend, is Norwegian Fish Oil, made by Carlson, in a liquid supplement with natural lemon or orange flavors, which makes it easy to take a high dose without having to take many pills.

> ➡ **What to do:** Take two teaspoons, twice a day. Pure DHA is also available in capsules, but is more expensive for a comparable dose.

▶ Magnesium

Magnesium reduces excitotoxicity and brain inflammation, improves blood flow to the brain, and raises levels of our chief internal antioxidant, glutathione, in brain cells. For best absorption, use a slow-release version of magnesium malate, such as Magnesium w/SRT, made by Jigsaw Health. Two caplets contain 250 mg. L-Threonate enters the brain better and comes in a 2,000 mg per capsule dose. I would recommend using both.

> ➡ **What to do:** Take two caplets of the Jigsaw brand, twice a day with meals. Take two capsules of the magnesium-L-threonate two to three times a day.

▶ Curcumin

An extract from the curry spice turmeric, curcumin is therapeutic because it is well established as a powerful anti-inflammatory. Most important, it can calm specific types of immune cells in the brain, called microglia and macrophages, which are related to neurodegeneration. It also raises brain levels of a neurotransmitter called acetylcholine, which improves memory and calms brain inflammation. And, curcumin reduces aluminum toxicity. For best absorption, use CurcumaSorb, made by Pure Encapsulations, which contains 250 mg per capsule.

> ➥ **What to do:** Take one capsule of CurcumaSorb, three times a day with meals. Because it has a high degree of safety, even in very large doses, you can increase the dose to 500 mg (two capsules), three times a day with meals. If you use a different product, for best absorption, I recommend opening capsules and mixing the contents with a teaspoon of coconut oil or extra virgin olive oil, taking the mixture, and then drinking some water. This is messy but important, as dry, powdered curcumin in many supplements is typically not well absorbed.

▶ Luteolin

This is a flavonoid found in several plants, such as celery and artichoke. A number of studies have shown that it powerfully reduces brain inflammation by quieting key immune cells, the microglia and macrophages, and immunoexcitotoxicity.

> ➥ **What to do:** Take 100 mg, three times a day with meals. After one week, the dose can be increased to 300 mg, three times a day with meals.

▶ Acetyl-L-Carnitine and Vinpocetine

A specific form of carnitine, acetyl-L-carnitine is a natural compound that has been shown to enhance brain function. It improves the connections between brain cells, reduces inflammation and excitotoxicity, and improves brain energy production. Vinpocetine is extracted from the periwinkle plant. It raises brain dopamine levels, improves blood flow in the brain, is a powerful anti-inflammatory, and has great potential to reduce neurodegeneration in both Alzheimer's and Parkinson's. A specific combination of these, Cresceo-ALC, made by Medix Select, contains 1,500 mg of acetyl-L-carnitine and 30 mg of vinpocetine in two capsules.

> ➡ **What to do:** Take one Cresceo-ALC capsule, twice a day with meals. The maximum dose is one capsule, three times a day with meals.

▶ Gastrodin

Studies of gastrodin, an extract from a Chinese herb called Gastrodia elata, show that it may relieve depression and anxiety by reducing brain inflammation and excitotoxicity. And, it protects brain stem cells, which reverses shrinkage of the hippocampal area of the brain and protects memory.

> ➡ **What to do:** Take 300 mg, once a day for a week, and then take the same amount twice a day.

▶ Niacinamide

Also called vitamin B3, niacinamide plays a major role in energy production by all cells, including brain cells.

> ➡ **What to do:** The usual dose is 500 mg, two to three times a day with meals.

▶ Multivitamin/Mineral

People at risk of neurodegenerative disorders need adequate intake of all of the major vitamins and minerals. Iron should not be in your supplement, as in most cases of neurodegenerative diseases we see excess iron in the brain and spinal cord. A good product should include all of the B vitamins in an absorbable form, such as the "5-methyltetrahydrofolate" form of folic acid, multiple forms of natural vitamin E, some vitamin C, and the trace minerals.

➡️ **What to do:** Follow directions for the product you choose.

▶ **Methylcobalamin (vitamin B12)**
This is the most absorbable and beneficial form of vitamin B12, which is essential for energy production in the brain but often in short supply among older people. I prefer a sublingual form, which dissolves under the tongue.

➡️ **What to do:** Take 10,000 mcg a day of a sublingual form.

▶ **Hyperbaric Oxygen Therapy (HBOT)**
Several studies have shown improvement in aged-related memory loss as a result of HBOT treatments. This is not surprising, as the disorder is caused by inflammation and excitotoxicity, and HBOT reduces both.

Stroke Prevention

A stroke stops oxygen and nutrients from reaching the brain and causes brain cells to die. The result can be lost ability to walk, talk, control muscles, and sometimes complete paralysis of one side of the body. There are two main types of strokes: 87 percent of strokes are ischemic, in which a blood vessel is blocked, and others are hemorrhagic, in which there is bleeding in the brain. In both cases, atherosclerosis, also called a hardening of the arteries, is the underlying mechanism.

Before a full-blown stroke occurs, there are usually mild, brief symptoms, such as sudden numbness of one side of the face or an arm, dizzy spells, confusion that lasts for just a minute, heaviness of an arm or leg, and problems with speech, such as attempting to say a word or repeating words over and over. Taking an aspirin when symptoms first occur can prevent most strokes, but it is important to then see your doctor for a proper workup, as soon as possible.

⌬ Conventional Treatment

A stroke caused by a blocked artery is treated with anti-coagulant drugs. The bleeding in a hemorrhagic stroke may be stopped with intravenous drugs, a catheter, or with surgery. Depending on the severity of the stroke, rehabilitation may require physical therapy. To prevent another stroke, or to prevent a first stroke in people at risk, medications are used to treat risk factors, such as high blood pressure, or to control diabetes. Drugs that thin the blood may be prescribed.

👍 My Recommendations

Contrary to popular wisdom, cholesterol does not cause strokes—chronic inflammation does. Inflammation leads to atherosclerosis, a build-up of plaque in the inner lining of arteries. Plaque impedes blood flow, and when the plaque ruptures, it can form a clot that creates a blockage. The cause of this inflammation varies and there may be more than one trigger, including chronic bacterial or viral infections; exposure to toxic metals, such as lead, mercury, cadmium, or aluminum; a poor diet; stress; high blood pressure; environmental pollutants such as exhaust fumes; and autoimmune diseases. Treating existing medical conditions will reduce stroke risk and, should a stroke occur, improve the quality of recovery.

By reducing inflammation, we can reduce atherosclerosis and risk for stroke. Diet, which is most critical, and anti-inflammatory supplements offer the best course to achieve this goal. See chapter 1 for the

ARE YOU AT RISK FOR STROKE?
Chronic inflammation, which is not observable in daily life, underlies strokes. These are some observable risk factors:
• High blood pressure
• Smoking
• Poor diet
• Lack of physical activity
• Obesity, especially in the abdomen
• Atrial fibrillation
• Taking birth control pills or steroids
• Family history of stroke
• Migraine headaches
• Diabetes

anti-inflammatory diet and lifestyle in more detail, but these are the key points:

- Eat and drink vegetables (recipe is in chapter 3)
- Eat the right meats
- Know your fats
- Drink purified water and white and green teas
- Avoid trans fats
- Avoid sugar
- Minimize starchy carbohydrates
- Avoid fluoride
- Maintain healthy teeth
- Exercise regularly
- Avoid prolonged, excessive stress

What most people find surprising is that sugar, so copious in today's food supply, is the big driver of atherosclerosis. Despite what your doctor may have told you, and you will quite likely continue to hear, saturated fat is not the bad guy. While I'm not advocating overindulgence in fatty foods, I can't emphasize enough that sugar is the culprit, and it has many variations.

High fructose corn syrup, for example, is in just about any kind of packaged or processed food. It's found in soups, sauces, savory breads and buns, condiments, frozen meals, processed meats, and many "healthy" foods, such as flavored yogurts. Because this sweetener has been criticized, some food products are now touted for containing "real cane sugar." That's still sugar, and it doesn't make them any healthier. An overabundance of starch has the same effect, because starch is turned into sugar in the human body.

Natural Supplements

As well as eating an anti-inflammatory diet, it is important to take a multivitamin for essential vitamins and minerals. In addition, many plant extracts and nutrient compounds have very powerful anti-inflammatory and antioxidant properties that reduce atherosclerosis. These are some of the best ones.

▸ Curcumin

Studies show that curcumin, an extract from the curry spice turmeric, is one of the most powerful anti-inflammatory compounds and can dramatically reduce atherosclerosis. And, it has a slight anticoagulant effect, which helps reduce heart attacks. CurcumaSorb, made by Pure Encapsulations, contains 250 mg per capsule and is a well-absorbed product.

- **What to do:** Take one to two capsule of CurcumaSorb, three times a day with meals.

▸ Quercetin

Another powerful anti-inflammatory and antioxidant, in animal studies, quercetin has produced significant prevention of atherosclerosis. Use a well-absorbed product such as Quercenase, made by Thorne Research.

- **What to do:** Take one capsule of Quercenase, which contains 250 mg of quercetin, three times a day with meals.

▸ Luteolin

Several studies have shown that Luteolin inhibits atherosclerosis through a number of mechanisms. It calms special white blood cells, called macrophages, which play a major role in atherosclerosis. A good product is Luteolin Complex, made by Swanson Health Products, which contains 100 mg per capsule.

- **What to do:** Take two capsules of Luteolin Complex, three times a day with meals.

▸ Apigenin

Found in celery, parsley, and apples, it is a powerful anti-inflammatory and inhibits atherosclerosis. A good product is

Apigenin, made by Swanson Health Products, which contains 50 mg per capsule.

➡ **What to do:** Take two capsules, three times a day with meals.

▶ Aged Garlic Extract

This is a special form of garlic. A number of human studies have shown that it not only reduces atherosclerosis, but might reverse it as well. The product, which is odorless, is called Kyolic Aged Garlic Extract, made by Wakunaga.

➡ **What to do:** Take one capsule of Kyolic Aged Garlic Extract 100% Vegetarian Cardiovascular Formula 100, twice a day with meals.

▶ Mixed Tocopherols and Tocotrienols (Vitamin E)

Natural vitamin E is not one single compound but a combination, grouped into subtypes called tocopherols and tocotrienols. Together, they offer rather powerful inhibition of atherosclerosis.

➡ **What to do:** Take 400 IU of mixed tocopherols and 50 mg of mixed tocotrienols, twice a day, with or without meals.

▶ Magnesium

Magnesium reduces inflammation, raises levels of our major internal antioxidant, glutathione, helps to keep arteries flexible, and improves blood flow, even through the smallest blood vessels, called arterioles and capillaries. For optimum absorption, take either magnesium citrate or malate. A slow-release form is best, such as Magnesium w/SRT, made by Jigsaw Health.

➡ **What to do:** Take two slow-release tablets, twice a day with meals.

▶ Hyperbaric Oxygen Therapy (HBOT)

A number of animal and human studies have looked at the effect of HBOT on stroke damage in the brain. Most demonstrate better long-term improvement with HBOT treatments. Studies that show little or no effect are usually poorly done or use improper techniques, such as inadequate atmospheric pressure, insufficient levels of oxygen, or an insufficient number of treatments.

CHAPTER 16

Mouth, Eyes, and Ears

» Cataracts
» Dry Eyes
» Glaucoma
» Gum Disease
» Macular Degeneration, Age-Related

» Mouth Ulcers
» Tinnitus
» Vision Health

Cataracts

Cataracts affect 22 million Americans after age 40, and by age 80 one in two either have cataracts or have had surgery to correct the condition. Cataracts manifest as a clouding of the lens, creating a foggy view. The lens of the eye, which works much like a camera, is made mostly of water and protein. The protein is designed to keep the lens clear but can start to form clumps that form a film or cloud. Initially, a cataract may affect only part of an individual's visual field but as it gets bigger, a greater part of the lens is affected, making it more difficult to see.

Conventional Treatment

Regular eye check-ups can detect cataracts and glasses can help to improve vision. Sunglasses and wide-brimmed hats can also help by reducing glare and may help to slow progression of the disease.

WHAT INCREASES RISK FOR CATARACTS?

Although age itself is considered a key risk factor, these also increase risk:

- Diabetes
- Obesity
- High blood pressure
- Smoking
- Eye injury or surgery earlier in life
- Family history of cataracts
- Drinking excessive alcohol
- Excessive exposure to sunlight
- Exposure to radiation from x-rays or during cancer treatment
- Taking corticosteroid medications for long periods

Bright lighting and magnifying lenses can help to improve vision indoors. Surgery is the only medical treatment and is usually done only when cataracts are significantly interfering with an individual's life. For ways to prevent or reverse type 2 diabetes, which increases risk for cataracts, see the section "Diabetes, Type 2" in chapter 14.

👍 My Recommendations

An anti-inflammatory diet, such as the one described in chapter 1, is very important because the progressive damage within the eye is related to high levels of inflammation. Excitotoxicity, described in chapter 2, is the other major trigger and needs to be reduced for prevention and slowing progression of any eye disease. An interaction between inflammation and excitotoxicity, which I call immunoexcitotoxicity, damages the neurons in the retina and this results in a loss of visual acuity. In a sense, this is good news because it means there is more we can do to prevent vision loss.

In a nutshell, an anti-inflammatory diet means avoiding inflammatory vegetable fats, such as corn, safflower, sunflower, peanut, corn, canola, and soybean oils, increasing your intake of the omega-3 oils found in fish, eating at least five to ten servings of fruits and vegetables daily, and avoiding sugar, especially high fructose corn syrup. One should also avoid all fluoride and aluminum, found in regular drinking water in many areas.

To protect the eyes, limit time spent looking at the screen of a computer or other electronic devices and wear UV-blocking sunglasses when outdoors. And, be aware that steroid drugs can cause cataracts.

🐇 Natural Supplements

▶ N-acetylcarnosine Eye Drops

Several studies have shown that in the case of cataracts, these eye drops can correct clouding of the lens in a significant number of people. Initially, they can cause some stinging of the eyes.

➡ **What to do:** Use per product directions.

▶ Lutein and Zeaxanthin

For eye health, these are some of the most important nutrients, as the retina contains very high levels of lutein and some zeaxanthin. Both protect it and are critical for good vision. Spinach and kale are excellent food sources of both.

➡ **What to do:** Lutein and zeaxanthin are combined in some supplements. Look for at least 20 mg of lutein per capsule in a product such as Synergistic Eye Formula Lutein & Zeaxanthin, made by Swanson Health Products. Take one capsule a day with food. For serious retinal disorders, take one capsule twice a day.

▶ Curcumin

An extract from the curry spice turmeric, curcumin has powerful anti-inflammatory properties, is a potent antioxidant, blocks immunoexcitotoxicity in the retina, and stimulates growth of junctions between cells in the retina, which improves vision. I recommend a well-absorbed form, such as CurcumaSorb, made by Pure Encapsulations, which contains 250 mg of curcumin per capsule.

➡ **What to do:** Take one CurcumaSorb capsule, three times a day with meals.

▶ Quercetin

This is a plant compound that is a potent antioxidant with powerful anti-inflammatory properties. It protects the retina against immunoexcitotoxicity, described in chapter 2. I recommend a well-absorbed form called Quercenase, made by Thorne Research, which contains 250 mg per capsule.

> ➡ **What to do:** Take one capsule, three times a day with meals.

▶ Astaxanthin

A powerful antioxidant found in some algae, it gives salmon their pink color. Astaxanthin plays a major role in protecting the retina, and hence vision. Look for a natural form derived from microalgae that is grown in a controlled environment without toxins.

> ➡ **What to do:** Astaxanthin supplements most often contain 4 mg per softgel capsule. Take two capsules, two to three times a day with meals.

▶ Vinpocetine

This natural substance from the periwinkle plant has been shown to improve blood flow in the smaller vessels of the retina and to reduce inflammation and excitotoxicity.

> ➡ **What to do:** Higher doses can cause headaches, so I recommend starting with 5 mg a day for three days, with a meal, then increase the dose to 5 mg, three times a day with meals, for two weeks. Then, for serious retinal diseases, the dose can be increased to 20 mg a day.

▶ N-Acetyl Cysteine (NAC)

NAC is a compound that safely increases levels of glutathione in the cells of the retina (and the rest of our bodies) and protects the lens of the eye.

> ➡ **What to do:** Take 750 mg, twice a day with meals. Taking NAC on an empty stomach can cause severe cramping.

▶ Vitamin C

Vitamin C is a powerful antioxidant. It's important to take a buffered form, which is gentle on the stomach and not acidic, such as Lypo-Spheric Vitamin C, made by LivOn Labs. It comes in packets of 1,000 mg, which are mixed with water or juice, and is highly absorbable.

➤ **What to do:** Take 1,000 mg, three times a day between meals. High-dose vitamin C dramatically increases iron absorption from food and, if taken with meals, can produce iron overload.

▶ Magnesium

The mineral reduces inflammation, raises levels of glutathione, one of our chief internal antioxidants, and improves blood flow. It's important to take only the citrate or malate forms of magnesium, as other forms are not as well absorbed and can cause diarrhea at lower doses. The best form is slow-release, such as Magnesium w/ SRT, made by Jigsaw Health, which contains 500 mg in two tablets.

➤ **What to do:** Take two tablets of Magnesium w/SRT, twice a day with meals.

▶ Fish Oil

A pure, good-quality fish oil supplement will increase anti-inflammatory omega-3 fats in the diet. A high-dose liquid supplement, such as Norwegian Fish Oil, made by Carlson, is easy to use and doesn't require taking multiple capsules.

➤ **What to do:** Take one to two teaspoons of the liquid oil by Carlson, twice a day.

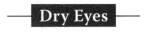

Dry Eyes

The corneas of the eyes contain no blood vessels and therefore depend on a regular bath of tears to keep the surface of the eyes moist. When our bodies don't make enough of that lubricating fluid, technically called "tears," or it isn't the right consistency, eye problems can develop. Most often, lack of lubrication on the surface of the eye causes discomfort and altered vision, which can range from mild irritation to more severe inflammation, with intense eye pain and severely impaired vision.

With the frequent use of smartphones and other electronic devices, dry eye is a growing problem among younger people and children, but generally, its incidence increases with age. One of the problems with electronic devices is that people tend to blink a lot less. Dry eye can also be a side effect of medications or corneal surgery to correct vision. While in most cases this post-operative problem subsides in a few weeks or months, in some, it can linger.

SYMPTOMS OF DRY EYE
Most symptoms relate to a feeling of dryness, but sometimes, the condition can trigger overproduction of the watery substance we normally think of as tears, causing watery eyes. Symptoms may include:
• Red, irritated, or burning eyes
• Eyes that feel scratchy
• Feeling that something is in your eye
• Slowed reading speed
• Blurry vision
• Difficulty looking at a computer screen

Recent studies indicate that dry eye may, in fact, be a form of autoimmune reaction, with elevated levels of inflammatory substances, called cytokines, within the cornea. Aging is the most common contributing factor, particularly among postmenopausal women. Certain medications, such as antihistamines, diuretics, some antidepressants, and beta blockers can also increase one's risk. Dry eye is also associated with certain diseases, such as diabetes, Sjogren's syndrome, glaucoma, and sarcoidosis, an inflammatory disorder. A number of tests can be done by ophthalmologists to diagnose the cause of the problem. In 60 percent of cases, there are no symptoms.

Conventional Treatment

Many people use over-the-counter eye drops to improve lubrication and reduce redness and pain. Several are quite helpful in relieving symptoms but not curing the basic problem. You should avoid eye drops that contain benzalkonium chloride as a preservative.

Eye doctors may prescribe different types of eye drops. In some situations, they may use special devices to unblock glands and ducts that supply fluid, or to prevent fluid from draining too rapidly. For people who wear contacts, different drops may be needed. Some newer medications aim to reduce inflammation or suppress immune-system reactions in the eyes, but can lead to complications. Where dry eye may be a side effect of medications taken to treat other conditions, these need to be reviewed and adjusted.

👍 My Recommendations

It is important to avoid the obvious things, such as cigarette smoke and excessive use of heaters and air conditioners. It helps to use humidifiers and drink plenty of water each day. When working on a computer for long periods, look away from the screen as often as possible and remember to blink frequently. It is also helpful to turn down the brightness of the screen.

Lack of omega-3 oils in the diet, found in fish, is one of the most common deficiencies leading to dry eye. The DHA component of fish oil is especially important. In fact, special topical DHA drops have been shown to significantly improve dry eye following laser eye surgery because they help to restore fine nerves that are damaged during the surgery.

Studies show that, for most people, taking fish oil improves the quality of the tears and healing of the corneas. Eating an anti-inflammatory diet, described in chapter 1, will also help.

🐇 Natural Supplements

▶ Fish Oil

I recommend a pure, good-quality product with a high DHA component, such as a liquid Norwegian Fish Oil, made by Carlson. There are also supplements that contain only DHA.

> ➡ **What to do:** Take one to two teaspoons of the liquid oil by Carlson, twice a day. Higher doses may be needed for severe dry eye, such as a tablespoon, twice a day. If you

take only DHA in capsules, I suggest taking 200 mg, two to three times a day.

▶ Curcumin

Since dry eye is an inflammatory condition, anti-inflammatory plant compounds, such as flavonoids in curcumin, can be of benefit. Studies have shown that curcumin lowers the levels of inflammation in tears and improves their quality. I recommend using a product that is well absorbed, such as CurcumaSorb, made by Pure Encapsulations, which contains 250 mg in one capsule.

➡ **What to do:** Take one capsule of CurcumaSorb, three times a day with meals.

▶ Grape Seed Extract

This extract has been shown to reduce several types of inflammatory substances in the human body and calms autoimmune reactions. It should help dry eye.

➡ **What to do:** Take 500 mg, three times a day, with or without meals. If you don't like taking pills, you can open up capsules and mix the contents in a glass of water or blueberry juice.

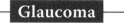

Glaucoma

Glaucoma is a leading cause of vision loss in the United States, second only to age-related macular degeneration. Its exact mechanics within the eye can vary somewhat, as there are several subtypes of the disease. Eye pressure that is higher than normal plays a role in some, but not all cases, but the common thread is damage to the optic nerve that carries visual information to the brain. Loss of peripheral vision is an earlier symptom, followed by greater vision loss, which can progress slowly or more rapidly.

⚕ Conventional Treatment

Glaucoma can be treated with medications in the form of pills or eye drops and, in some cases, with surgery. Many people who are prescribed eye drops stop using them, either because of inconvenience or side effects. Regular physical activity that improves the health of the heart—the type that increases heart rate during exercise—can help to prevent excessive pressure in the eye, and may help to reduce risk for glaucoma.

> **GLAUCOMA FACTS**
>
> According to the American Academy of Ophthalmology:
>
> - In the United States, glaucoma affects more than 2.2 million people after age 40
> - Its incidence increases with age
> - By 2020, glaucoma is expected to affect 3.3 million Americans
> - About half of those affected don't know they have the disease

👍 My Recommendations

An anti-inflammatory diet, such as the one described in chapter 1, is very important because the progressive damage within the eye is related to high levels of inflammation. Excitotoxicity, described in chapter 2, is the other major trigger and needs to be reduced for prevention and slowing progression of any eye disease. As an example, glaucoma is generally believed to be caused by pressure in the eye but newer evidence shows that this may not be the major culprit. Rather, an interaction between inflammation and excitotoxicity, which I call immunoexcitotoxicity, damages the neurons in the retina and this results in a loss of visual acuity. In a sense, this is good news because it means there is more we can do to prevent vision loss.

In a nutshell, an anti-inflammatory diet means avoiding inflammatory vegetable fats, such as corn, safflower, sunflower, peanut, canola, and soybean oils, increasing your intake of the omega-3 oils found in fish, eating at least five to ten servings of fruits and vegetables daily, and avoiding sugar, especially high fructose corn syrup. One should also avoid all fluoride and aluminum, found in regular drinking water in many areas.

To protect the eyes, limit time spent looking at the screen of a computer or other electronic devices and wear UV-blocking sunglasses when outdoors.

🐇 Natural Supplements

▶ Lutein and Zeaxanthin

For eye health, these are some of the most important nutrients, as the retina contains very high levels of lutein and some zeaxanthin. Both protect it and are critical for good vision. Spinach and kale are excellent foods sources of both.

> ➡ **What to do:** Lutein and zeaxanthin are combined in some supplements. Look for at least 20 mg of lutein per capsule, in a product such as Synergistic Eye Formula Lutein & Zeaxanthin, made by Swanson Health Products. Take one capsule a day with food. For serious retinal disorders, take one capsule twice a day.

▶ Curcumin

An extract from the curry spice turmeric, curcumin has powerful anti-inflammatory properties, is a potent antioxidant, blocks immunoexcitotoxicity in the retina, and stimulates growth of junctions between cells in the retina, which improves vision. I recommend a well-absorbed form, such as CurcumaSorb, made by Pure Encapsulations, which contains 250 mg of curcumin per capsule.

> ➡ **What to do:** Take one CurcumaSorb capsule, three times a day with meals.

▶ Quercetin

This is a plant compound that is a potent antioxidant with powerful anti-inflammatory properties. It protects the retina against immunoexcitotoxicity, described in chapter 2. I recommend a well-absorbed form called Quercenase, made by Thorne Research, which contains 250 mg per capsule.

➡ **What to do:** Take one capsule, three times a day with meals.

▶ Astaxanthin

A powerful antioxidant found in some algae, it gives salmon their pink color. Astaxanthin plays a major role in protecting the retina, and hence vision. Look for a natural form derived from microalgae that is grown in a controlled environment without toxins.

➡ **What to do:** Astaxanthin supplements most often contain 4 mg per softgel capsule. Take two capsules, two to three times a day with meals.

▶ Vinpocetine

This natural substance from the periwinkle plant has been shown to improve blood flow in the smaller vessels of the retina and to reduce inflammation and excitotoxicity.

➡ **What to do:** Higher doses can cause headaches, so I recommend starting with 5 mg a day for three days, with a meal, then increase the dose to 5 mg, three times a day with meals, for two weeks. Then, for serious retinal diseases, the dose can be increased to 20 mg a day.

▶ N-Acetyl Cysteine (NAC)

NAC is a compound that safely increases levels of glutathione in the cells of the retina (and the rest of our bodies) and protects the lens of the eye. People with glaucoma have very low levels of glutathione in their eyes.

➡ **What to do:** Take 750 mg, twice a day with meals. Taking NAC on an empty stomach can cause severe cramping.

▶ Vitamin C

Several studies have shown that vitamin C lowers pressure in the eyes in cases of glaucoma and that this can occur very rapidly. It does not lower pressure in healthy eyes. Vitamin C is also a powerful antioxidant. It's important to take a buffered form, which is gentle on the stomach and not acidic, such as Lypo-Spheric Vitamin C, made by LivOn Labs. It comes in packets of 1,000 mg, which are mixed with water or juice, and is highly absorbable.

> ➡ **What to do:** Take 1,000 mg, three times a day between meals. High-dose vitamin C dramatically increases iron absorption from food and, if taken with meals, can produce iron overload.

▶ Ginkgo Biloba

This plant extract has been shown to improve blood flow in the optic nerve and retina and to significantly improve vision in people with glaucoma. The supplement should contain a standardized extract, such as Ginkgo 50, made by Pure Encapsulations. It contains 160 mg per capsule.

> ➡ **What to do:** Take one capsule of Ginkgo 50, once or twice a day with meals. Ginkgo has anti-coagulant properties and should not be taken with aspirin or blood-thinning medications.

▶ Magnesium

The mineral reduces inflammation, raises levels of glutathione, one of our chief internal antioxidants, and improves blood flow. It's important to take only the citrate or malate forms of magnesium, as other forms are not as well absorbed and can cause diarrhea at lower doses. The best form is slow-release, such as Magnesium w/SRT, made by Jigsaw Health, which contains 500 mg in two tablets.

> ➡ **What to do:** Take two tablets of Magnesium w/SRT, twice a day with meals.

▶ Fish Oil

A pure, good-quality fish oil supplement will increase anti-inflammatory omega-3 fats in the diet. A high-dose liquid supplement, such as Norwegian Fish Oil, made by Carlson, is easy to use and doesn't require taking multiple capsules.

➽ **What to do:** Take one to two teaspoons of the liquid oil by Carlson, twice a day.

▶ Hyperbaric Oxygen Therapy (HBOT)

Most eye disorders, especially those that involve the retina, are improved by HBOT. This is because most of these retinal diseases are triggered by excitotoxins, and HBOT reduces levels of excitotoxins and inflammation. Glaucoma has traditionally been considered to be a disease driven by high pressure in the eye but is now known to be a disorder triggered by excitotoxins.

Gum Disease

The most common reason for tooth loss—gum disease—affects half of Americans after age 30 and 70 percent after age 65. The technical term, "periodontal disease," stems from two Greek words: *peri*, for "around," and *odon*, for "tooth." Periodontal disease is a chronic inflammation of the tissue around the teeth. As it progresses, gums become destroyed, pockets form around teeth, and eventually there is a loss of underlying bone that supports the teeth. In addition, inflammation and bacteria in pockets around teeth are associated with other inflammatory conditions, such as heart disease, strokes, atherosclerosis, and diabetes, and may contribute to or even precipitate neurodegenerative diseases, such as Alzheimer's and Parkinson's.

SIGNS OF GUM DISEASE
One or more of these indicate some degree of gum disease:
• Red, swollen, or tender gums
• Blood on your tooth brush
• Sensitivity to hot or cold foods or drinks
• Shrinking gums, exposing the roots of teeth
• Discomfort or pain when chewing
• Loose teeth

ᗇ Conventional Treatment

Brushing after each meal and flossing at least once each day, along with regular cleanings at the dentist, can help to preserve a healthy mouth throughout life. Where gum disease has developed, deep cleaning at the dentist, under the gums of each tooth, reduces hidden bacteria and inflammation. In severe cases, this may require surgery to reach deep pockets around teeth. The same treatments also smooth the roots of teeth, improving the attachment of gums and helping to preserve teeth. To reduce harmful bacteria in pockets around teeth, dentists sometimes prescribe antibiotics.

👍 My Recommendations

While not commonly discussed, diet can play a major role in health of the teeth and gums. While a diet high in sugar is often discussed as a cause for tooth decay and gum disease, the role played by eating fresh vegetables and calcium-containing foods, and avoiding fluoride, is not. Fluoride was sold to the public as a tooth-decay preventative, but numerous studies have shown that it destroys the outer layer of the tooth, which is the hardest part, and this increases tooth decay. In addition, it produces an erosive effect that leaves holes in the surface of the tooth along with a brownish discoloration, called dental fluorosis. In areas of the country with fluoridated drinking water supplies, the incidence of dental fluorosis can be as high as 40 percent.

You should avoid smoking and all other forms of tobacco and excessive use of alcohol. Alcohol-containing and fluoridated mouthwashes should be avoided, as should fluoride-containing toothpaste. A diet high in vegetables and low in red meats will promote dental health. Cheese, because of its high calcium content, has been shown to reduce cavities. Calcium supplements can have the same beneficial effects. Children should not be given candied supplements of ascorbic acid (vitamin C) as they can cause erosion of teeth.

Acid reflux disease (GERD), experienced as heartburn, can also result in erosion of the teeth's enamel and should be corrected. Taking two capsules of DGL plus, made by Pure Encapsulations, just before bedtime will help protect against the acid reflux. (For more details, see the "Heartburn" section in chapter 9, "Digestion.") Regular brushing with a non-fluoride toothpaste and flossing at least twice a day, especially before bedtime, will significantly reduce tooth decay and gum disease.

🐰 Natural Supplements

Several supplements can be beneficial for both teeth and gums. Like all tissues, gums depend upon an adequate supply of vitamins and minerals. Specific nutrients, special types of oils, and plant extracts are antibacterial and antiviral and can help ward off tooth decay and gum disease.

▶ Coconut Oil

It has a powerful antibacterial effect and can improve gum health, if used correctly.

➡ **What to do:** Once a day, put a teaspoon of coconut oil in your mouth and swish it around, as you would mouthwash. Do this for about two minutes, then either swallow it or spit it out.

▶ Coenzyme Q10 (CoQ10)

Studies have shown that CoQ10 can significantly reduce periodontal disease. Swallowing a pill will help but getting it onto your gums is much more effective, and is a very good way to treat severe gum disease.

➡ **What to do:** Mix powdered CoQ10 (from a capsule) with a teaspoon of extra virgin olive oil or coconut oil and swish it around your mouth, coating the gums. Hold this solution in your mouth for two minutes and then swallow it. To wash down the oil, you can also swallow a small amount of water, but after that, do not drink any liquids for about five minutes.

▶ White, Green, and Chamomile Teas

There are many beneficial compounds, called flavonoids, in various plants, and teas made from these can deliver therapeutic nutrients directly to your gums. White and green teas have anti-inflammatory and antibacterial compounds, and chamomile tea is a rich source of apigenin, which strongly promotes gum health.

➡ **What to do:** Make it a habit to drink at least two cups of white, green, and/or chamomile tea each day.

Macular Degeneration, Age-Related

Age-related macular degeneration is the leading cause of vision loss in the United States, more so than cataracts and glaucoma combined. It affects more than 2 million Americans age 50 and older. The condition is a deterioration of the macula, the central portion of the retina, which enables us to focus on the central portion of our field of vision, essential for driving, reading, recognizing faces, and seeing detail.

MACULAR DEGENERATION FACTS

Risk for macular degeneration is higher among:

- People with a family history of the disease
- Those age 55 and older
- Caucasians
- Smokers–smoking doubles the risk

As the disease progresses, people experience wavy or blurred vision and eventually may completely lose central vision.

🔷 Conventional Treatment

There is no effective medical treatment for age-related macular degeneration, but a large clinical trial found that progression of the disease can be delayed with this combination of dietary supplements, taken daily: vitamin C (500 mg), vitamin E (400 IU), zinc oxide (80 mg), copper as cupric oxide (2 mg), lutein (10 mg), and zeaxanthin (2 mg). The combination is found in some eye-health formulas.

👍 My Recommendations

An anti-inflammatory diet, such as the one described in chapter 1, is very important because the progressive damage within the eye is related to high levels of inflammation. Excitotoxicity, described in chapter 2, is the other major trigger and needs to be reduced for prevention and slowing progression of any eye disease. An interaction between inflammation and excitotoxicity, which I call immunoexcitotoxicity, damages the neurons in the retina and this results in a loss of visual acuity. In a sense, this is good news because it means there is more we can do to prevent vision loss.

In a nutshell, an anti-inflammatory diet means avoiding inflammatory vegetable fats, such as corn, safflower, sunflower, peanut, canola, and soybean oils, increasing your intake of the omega-3 oils found in fish, eating at least five to ten servings of fruits and vegetables daily, and avoiding sugar, especially high fructose corn syrup. One should also avoid all fluoride and aluminum, found in regular drinking water in many areas.

To protect the eyes, limit time spent looking at the screen of a computer or other electronic devices and wear UV-blocking sunglasses when outdoors.

🦃 Natural Supplements

▶ Lutein and Zeaxanthin

For eye health, these are some of the most important nutrients, as the retina contains very high levels of lutein and some zeaxanthin. Both protect it and are critical for good vision. Spinach and kale are excellent foods sources of both.

> ➡ **What to do:** Lutein and zeaxanthin are combined in some supplements. Look for at least 20 mg of lutein per capsule,

in a product such as Synergistic Eye Formula Lutein & Zeaxanthin, made by Swanson Health Products. Take one capsule a day with food. For serious retinal disorders, one capsule can be taken twice a day.

▶ Curcumin

An extract from the curry spice turmeric, curcumin has powerful anti-inflammatory properties, is a potent antioxidant, blocks immunoexcitotoxicity in the retina, and stimulates growth of junctions between cells in the retina, which improves vision. I recommend a well-absorbed form, such as CurcumaSorb, made by Pure Encapsulations, which contains 250 mg of curcumin per capsule.

➡ **What to do:** Take one CurcumaSorb capsule, three times a day with meals.

▶ Quercetin

This is a plant compound that is a potent antioxidant with powerful anti-inflammatory properties. It protects the retina against immunoexcitotoxicity, described in chapter 2. I recommend a well-absorbed form called Quercenase, made by Thorne Research, which contains 250 mg per capsule.

➡ **What to do:** Take one capsule, three times a day with meals.

▶ Astaxanthin

A powerful antioxidant found in some algae, it gives salmon their pink color. Astaxanthin plays a major role in protecting the retina, and hence vision. Look for a natural form derived from microalgae that is grown in a controlled environment without toxins.

➡ **What to do:** Astaxanthin supplements most often contain 4 mg per softgel capsule. Take two capsules, two to three times a day with meals.

▶ Vinpocetine

This natural substance from the periwinkle plant has been shown to improve blood flow in the smaller vessels of the retina and to reduce inflammation and excitotoxicity.

➡ **What to do:** Higher doses can cause headaches, so I recommend starting with 5 mg a day for three days, with a meal, then increase the dose to 5 mg, three times a day with meals, for two weeks. Then, for serious retinal diseases, the dose can be increased to 20 mg a day.

▶ N-Acetyl Cysteine (NAC)

NAC is a compound that safely increases levels of glutathione in the cells of the retina (and the rest of our bodies) and protects the lens of the eye.

➡ **What to do:** Take 750 mg, twice a day with meals. Taking NAC on an empty stomach can cause severe cramping.

▶ Vitamin C

Vitamin C is a powerful antioxidant. It's important to take a buffered form, which is gentle on the stomach and not acidic, such as Lypo-Spheric Vitamin C, made by LivOn Labs. It comes in packets of 1,000 mg, which are mixed with water or juice, and is highly absorbable.

➡ **What to do:** Take 1,000 mg, three times a day between meals. High-dose vitamin C dramatically increases iron absorption from food and, if taken with meals, can produce iron overload.

▶ Magnesium

The mineral reduces inflammation, raises levels of glutathione, one of our chief internal antioxidants, and improves blood flow. It's important to take only the citrate or malate forms of magnesium, as other forms are not as well absorbed and can cause diarrhea at lower doses. The best form is slow-release, such as

Magnesium w/SRT, made by Jigsaw Health, which contains 500 mg in two tablets.

➧ **What to do:** Take two tablets of Magnesium w/SRT, twice a day with meals.

▶ **Fish Oil**

A pure, good-quality fish oil supplement will increase anti-inflammatory omega-3 fats in the diet. A high-dose liquid supplement, such as Norwegian Fish Oil, made by Carlson, is easy to use and doesn't require taking multiple capsules.

➧ **What to do:** Take one to two teaspoons of the liquid oil by Carlson, twice a day.

▶ **Hyperbaric Oxygen Therapy (HBOT)**

HBOT can deliver benefits to those with age-related macular degeneration by delivering more oxygen to the retina and improving blood flow to the eye. HBOT also stimulates the formation of healthy microvessels and reduces excitoxicity that damages the eye.

—— Mouth Ulcers ——

Mouth ulcers are painful sores along the gum line, inside lips, or in other parts of the mouth. In most cases, they are the result of reactivation of the herpes simplex virus, which lies dormant in special ganglion cells in nerves of the head. These ulcers can develop after a minor injury, such as biting your cheek or accidentally piercing the skin with a toothpick. The injury activates the sleeping virus.

Conventional Treatment

Where mouth ulcers persist or recur, treatment would depend upon the diagnosis of the cause. A dentist or doctor may do a biopsy or blood tests as part of an exam and would need to consider an individual's medical history for possible causes. These could include a herpes virus, other infections in the body, a dental abscess, and oral cancer, or the ulcers could be a reaction to a chemical additive in toothpaste, mouthwash, or food.

> **PREVENTION BASICS**
>
> Good dental habits can help prevent mouth ulcers by reducing the risk of infection in the mouth. However, brushing teeth too vigorously, especially with a hard or medium toothbrush, can injure tissues and trigger a sore. Brushing gently with a soft toothbrush twice a day, as well as flossing once daily, helps to prevent any type of infection in the mouth.

👍 My Recommendations

It's critical to avoid acid-generating foods, as blood acidity can wake up the herpes simplex virus and trigger ulcer formation. Foods to avoid include vinegar, ketchup, tomato sauces, large quantities of meat, and sugar. Vegetables are generally alkaline, so increasing your intake will keep the virus asleep. Good oral hygiene is also vital, as gum disease can activate the virus and hence mouth ulcers.

This is a simple way to rapidly neutralize the acid in your body and speed up healing of ulcers: mix a teaspoon of baking soda (sodium bicarbonate) in a small glass of water and drink it, two to three times a day. Silver (see below) is another remedy.

🏃 Natural Supplements

▶ Buffered Vitamin C

Vitamin C has powerful antiviral properties, but must be in a buffered form that is not acidic. If it is in the most common form of ascorbic acid, which is not buffered, it will increase acidity, which makes the ulcer problem worse. I recommend using a buffered form called Lypo-Spheric Vitamin C, made by LivOn Labs. It comes in packets of gel, each containing 1,000 mg of vitamin C, which you mix with water or juice. It prevents acidity and is absorbed more effectively than regular vitamin C.

➡ **What to do:** Take one packet of Lypo-Spheric Vitamin C, twice a day. Or, take another brand of buffered vitamin C, 1,000 mg, two to three times a day. Always take vitamin C on an empty stomach, as it increases iron absorption and taking it with food can lead to excess iron levels.

▶ **Silver Spray**

Silver works very well in quickly healing painful mouth ulcers. Use a silver spray containing 10 ppm bio-active silver, called Sovereign Silver, made by Natural Immunogenics.

➡ **What to do:** Spray the ulcerated area two or three times a day. Do not drink any liquids for 30 minutes after spraying.

Tinnitus

A ringing or other phantom noise in the ears, tinnitus can be fleeting or chronic and occurs more often among older people. It's estimated that one in five Americans experience it at some time. When it persists, tinnitus can significantly interfere with normal life but rather than being a disease, it is a symptom of something being awry. Often, it accompanies hearing loss, and can occur in one or both ears. Sometimes, tinnitus appears before any hearing loss becomes noticeable.

SOUNDS OF TINNITUS

Phantom noises that are the hallmark of tinnitus may have different sounds, including:

- Ringing
- Whining
- Squealing
- Hissing
- Roaring
- Buzzing
- Clicking

Conventional Treatment

Although it can be quite debilitating, tinnitus does not usually indicate a life-threatening situation. In rare instances, it can be an early sign of a benign brain tumor called an acoustic neuroma. Some of the common underlying conditions include buildup of ear wax, hearing loss, noise damage to the ear, reactions to a medication, or an infection in the middle ear. When these are treated, the tinnitus often disappears. Where it persists, devices that mask the sound can be helpful, and may be in a hearing aid or similar device worn in the ear. There are no medications designed to treat tinnitus, but sometimes antidepressants or antianxiety drugs are prescribed, although these pose risks and do not actually treat the tinnitus.

👍 My Recommendations

We tend to think of damage to the hearing nerves as the main cause of tinnitus, but studies also show that damage can be deep within the brain stem. In cases of prolonged tinnitus, most treatments fail, even the natural ones. However, natural supplements such as curcumin, resveratrol, quercetin, apigenin, and luteolin can help to prevent damage to the brain. See chapter 15, "Brain Health," especially the "Alzheimer's, Parkinson's, and ALS" section, for how to use these. The anti-inflammatory diet in chapter 1 also protects the brain.

A number of flavonoids, a class of beneficial compounds in plants, can protect the hearing nerve from damage by drugs, such as certain antibiotics and chemotherapy, and noise-induced hearing loss, especially if started as soon as the damage occurs. The two supplements below are sources of such flavonoids and have been shown to reduce tinnitus and improve hearing and brain health.

🐇 Natural Supplements

▶ Vinpocetine

This extract from the periwinkle plant contains antioxidants and has a number of beneficial effects on hearing, such as improved blood flow, reduced inflammation, and protection of delicate neurons within the brain stem. Studies found that when used within one week of a hearing injury, 50 percent of people who took vinpocetine experienced complete disappearance of tinnitus. Studies have also shown that, even if treatment was started long after a hearing injury, between 66 and 79 percent of people experienced a significant decrease in tinnitus.

> ➡ **What to do:** The dose varies from 5 mg, three times a day, to as high as 20 mg, three times a day, depending on the severity of the problem. I recommend starting with 5 mg, three times a day for a week, as the higher dose can cause headaches. Gradually increasing the dose will usually prevent such headaches.

▶ Ginkgo Biloba

Ginkgo, extracted from one of the oldest living trees, contains a number of beneficial compounds, including quercetin. It has powerful anti-inflammatory and antioxidant properties and improves blood flow. It is most effective when used right after onset of tinnitus. Ginkgo will slightly interfere with coagulation, about as much as an aspirin with the usual ginkgo dose (below), so I would not take it with anticoagulant medications. Purity is essential in ginkgo products. The supplement should contain a standardized extract, such as Ginkgo 50, made by Pure Encapsulations. It contains 160 mg per capsule.

> ➡ **What to do:** Take one to two capsules of Ginkgo 50 daily, with a meal. Some studies used a dose as high as 320 mg, twice a day.

▶ Hyperbaric Oxygen Therapy (HBOT)

Several studies have tested HBOT in people with either sudden hearing loss or tinnitus. In most patients, both hearing and tinnitus improved. The earlier the HBOT is used, the better the results.

Vision Health

Nearsightedness (seeing things well only if they are close) and farsightedness (seeing things well only when they are further away) are common with age and can be corrected with glasses. There is some evidence, and I firmly believe this, that constantly using glasses actually makes vision worse, but they are necessary, as poor vision can lead to falls and other accidents. When it comes to more severe vision loss, these eye diseases are the most common causes:

> **PRESERVING HEALTHY VISION**
>
> Protecting the eyes from undue damage can help to preserve vision. These can all help:
>
> - Eating a nutritious diet
> - Wearing sunglasses to protect against UV rays
> - When using an electronic device, regularly looking away from the screen to relax eyes
> - Not smoking
> - Wearing protective eyewear when there is risk of injury

- Cataracts manifest as a clouding of the lens, creating a foggy view.

- Glaucoma results in a loss of visual acuity, either rapidly or slowly.

- Age-related macular degeneration impairs sight in the center of our field of vision.

- Diabetic retinopathy, a complication of diabetes which damages small blood vessels in the eye, causes blurred or spotty vision and difficulty seeing well at night.

Conventional Treatment

Vision loss related to type 2 diabetes can be prevented by treating the diabetes and ideally by preventing the disease in the first place (see the section "Diabetes, Type 2"). Regular eye check-ups can detect eye diseases earlier and, although none have a cure, their progression can often be delayed. Cataracts are most often treated with surgery. Glaucoma can be treated with medications in the form of pills or eye drops and, in some cases, with surgery.

There is no effective medical treatment for age-related macular degeneration, but a large clinical trial found that progression of the disease can be delayed with this combination of dietary supplements, taken daily: vitamin C (500 mg), vitamin E (400 IU), zinc oxide (80 mg), copper as cupric oxide (2 mg), lutein (10 mg), and zeaxanthin (2 mg), which is found in some eye-health formulas. For ways to prevent or reverse type 2 diabetes, see the section "Diabetes, Type 2" in chapter 14.

👍 My Recommendations

An anti-inflammatory diet, such as the one described in chapter 1, is very important because the progressive damage within the eye is related to high levels of inflammation. Excitotoxicity, described in chapter 2, is the other major trigger and needs to be reduced for prevention and slowing progression of any eye disease. As an example, glaucoma is generally believed to be caused by pressure in the eye but newer evidence shows that this may not be the major culprit. Rather, an interaction between inflammation and excitotoxicity, which I call immunoexcitotoxicity, damages the neurons in the retina and this results in a loss of visual acuity. In a sense, this is good news because it means there is more we can do to prevent vision loss.

In a nutshell, an anti-inflammatory diet means avoiding inflammatory vegetable fats, such as corn, safflower, sunflower, peanut, canola, and soybean oils, increasing your intake of the omega-3 oils found in fish, eating at least five to ten servings of fruits and vegetables daily, and avoiding sugar, especially high fructose corn syrup. One should also avoid all fluoride and aluminum, found in regular drinking water in many areas.

To protect the eyes, limit time spent looking at the screen of a computer or other electronic devices and wear UV-blocking sunglasses when outdoors. And, be aware that steroid drugs can cause cataracts.

Natural Supplements

▶ N-acetylcarnosine Eye Drops

Several studies have shown that in the case of cataracts, these eye drops can correct clouding of the lens in a significant number of people. Initially, they can causes some stinging of the eyes.

➡ **What to do:** Use per product directions.

▶ Lutein and Zeaxanthin

For eye health, these are some of the most important nutrients, as the retina contains very high levels of lutein and some zeaxanthin. Both protect it and are critical for good vision. Spinach and kale are excellent foods sources of both.

➡ **What to do:** Lutein and zeaxanthin are combined in some supplements. Look for at least 20 mg of lutein per capsule, in a product such as Synergistic Eye Formula Lutein & Zeaxanthin, made by Swanson Health Products. Take one capsule a day with food. For serious retinal disorders, one capsule can be taken twice a day.

▶ Curcumin

An extract from the curry spice turmeric, curcumin has powerful anti-inflammatory properties, is a potent antioxidant, blocks immunoexcitotoxicity in the retina, and stimulates growth of junctions between cells in the retina, which improves vision. I recommend a well-absorbed form, such as CurcumaSorb, made by Pure Encapsulations, which contains 250 mg of curcumin per capsule.

➡ **What to do:** Take one CurcumaSorb capsule, three times a day with meals.

▶ Quercetin

This is a plant compound that is a potent antioxidant with powerful anti-inflammatory properties. It protects the retina against immunoexcitotoxicity, described in chapter 2. I recommend a well-absorbed form called Quercenase, made by Thorne Research, which contains 250 mg per capsule.

➡ **What to do:** Take one capsule, three times a day with meals.

▶ Astaxanthin

A powerful antioxidant found in some algae, it gives salmon their pink color. Astaxanthin plays a major role in protecting the retina, and hence vision. Look for a natural form derived from microalgae that is grown in a controlled environment without toxins.

➡ **What to do:** Astaxanthin supplements most often contain 4 mg per softgel capsule. Take two capsules, two to three times a day with meals.

▶ Vinpocetine

This natural substance from the periwinkle plant has been shown to improve blood flow in the smaller vessels of the retina and to reduce inflammation and excitotoxicity.

➡ **What to do:** Higher doses can cause headaches, so I recommend starting with 5 mg a day for three days, with a meal, then increase the dose to 5 mg, three times a day with meals, for two weeks. Then, for serious retinal diseases, the dose can be increased to 20 mg a day.

▶ N-Acetyl Cysteine (NAC)

NAC is a compound that safely increases levels of glutathione in the cells of the retina (and the rest of our bodies) and protects the lens of the eye. People with glaucoma have very low levels of glutathione in their eyes.

➠ **What to do:** Take 750 mg, twice a day with meals. Taking NAC on an empty stomach can cause severe cramping.

▶ Vitamin C

Several studies have shown that vitamin C lowers pressure in the eyes in cases of glaucoma, and that this can occur very rapidly. It does not lower pressure in healthy eyes. Vitamin C is also a powerful antioxidant. It's important to take a buffered form, which is gentle on the stomach and not acidic, such as Lypo-Spheric Vitamin C, made by LivOn Labs. It comes in packets of 1,000 mg, which are mixed with water or juice, and is highly absorbable.

➠ **What to do:** Take 1,000 mg, three times a day between meals. High-dose vitamin C dramatically increases iron absorption from food and, if taken with meals, can produce iron overload.

▶ Ginkgo Biloba

This plant extract has been shown to improve blood flow in the optic nerve and retina and to significantly improve vision in people with glaucoma. The supplement should contain a standardized extract, such as Ginkgo 50, made by Pure Encapsulations. It contains 160 mg per capsule.

➠ **What to do:** Take one capsule of Ginkgo 50, once or twice a day with meals. Ginkgo has anti-coagulant properties and should not be taken with aspirin or blood-thinning medications.

▶ Magnesium

The mineral reduces inflammation, raises levels of glutathione, one of our chief internal antioxidants, and improves blood flow. It's important to take only the citrate or malate forms of magnesium, as other forms are not as well absorbed and can cause diarrhea at lower doses. The best form is slow-release, such as

Magnesium w/SRT, made by Jigsaw Health, which contains 500 mg in two tablets.

➡ **What to do:** Take two tablets of Magnesium w/SRT, twice a day with meals.

▶ **Fish Oil**

A pure, good-quality fish oil supplement will increase anti-inflammatory omega-3 fats in the diet. A high-dose liquid supplement, such as Norwegian Fish Oil, made by Carlson, is easy to use and doesn't require taking multiple capsules.

➡ **What to do:** Take one to two teaspoons of the liquid oil by Carlson, twice a day.

Supplement Buying Guide

Supplements can be found in health food stores, natural supermarkets, specialty supplement stores, and online. In some cases, a specific product and brand are recommended, and these are all listed alphabetically below. Where no brand name is mentioned, there are typically many brands of products of that type that will work well. However, it is best to use good quality supplements from established companies. If you aren't familiar with a brand, check its website.

Understanding Supplement Labels

By law, supplement labels must contain a Supplement Facts panel, which lists nutrients and quantities of each, and Other Ingredients, which includes other components used in making a pill or capsule. In the Supplement Facts panel, this is what common abbreviations mean:

- mg: milligrams

- mcg: micrograms

- g: grams

- IU: International Units

- CFU: colony forming units (used for probiotics)

"% Daily Value" or "% DV" is listed next to the quantity of each nutrient or extract in the Supplement Facts panel. The Daily Value is established by the FDA as an amount that is considered adequate to prevent a deficiency of that nutrient. This is not the same thing as a therapeutic amount recommended for specific benefits, which is usually higher. For example, the Daily Value for vitamin C is 60 mg, but 1,000 mg daily, or more, is recommended in many sections of this book. Not every nutrient and plant extract has a Daily Value, in which case labels note that one has not been established.

Other Important Label Information

These are some other things to look for on any supplement label:

- An expiry or "best before" date. Always use the product before this date.

- Contact information for the manufacturer, in case you have questions or need to report a problem.

- In the list of Other Ingredients, make sure there are no artificial colors, artificial flavors, artificial sweeteners, or chemical preservatives.

- If you have any allergies or food intolerances, check if the product is free of these, for example, "gluten-free" if you don't tolerate gluten.

- In the case of tablets or capsules, check how many make up a serving, as the nutrient quantities are given per serving, which could be anywhere from one to six pills.

Specific Products and Brands

In all the sections of this book, where a specific product is named by brand, it has particular characteristics in the way it is formulated, making it a good choice. For example, a recommended vitamin C product may be easier to absorb and digest than others, and other brands may not deliver the exact same benefit.

Below is a list of all these, by product name and by the name of the vitamin, mineral, or plant extract. To make it easier to find, one product may be listed under more than one letter of the alphabet. For example, Lypo-Spheric Vitamin C is listed under "L" and again under "V" for "vitamin C." The names and websites of manufacturers are also included.

▶ **Acetyl-L-Carnitine with Vinpocetine**
Cresceo-ALC
Medix Select: www.medixselect.com

▶ **Activated B-Complex High Bioavailability Formula**
Swanson Health Products: www.swansonvitamins.com

▶ **Aged Garlic Extract**
Kyolic Aged Garlic Extract 100% Vegetarian
Cardiovascular Formula 100
Wakunaga: www.kyolic.com

▶ **Apigenin**
Swanson Health Products: www.swansonvitamins.com

▶ **B-Complex for Brain Aging**
Activated B-Complex High Bioavailability Formula
Swanson Health Products: www.swansonvitamins.com

▶ **B Vitamins**
B-Complex Plus
Pure Encapsulations: www.pureencapsulations.com

▶ **B Vitamins in a Multivitamin**
Extend Core
Vitamin Research Products: www.vrp.com

▶ **Baicalein**
Baicalin
LiftMode: www.liftmode.com

▶ **Berberine-500**
Thorne Research: www.thorne.com

▶ **Betatene**
Swanson Health Products: www.swansonvitamins.com

▶ **BioCell Collagen**
Collagen JS
Pure Encapsulations: www.pureencapsulations.com

▶ **Body Lotion**
Derma e Vitamin E Intensive Therapy Body Lotion
Derma e: www.dermae.com

▶ **Borage Oil (topical)**
Borage Therapy
Shikai: www.shikai.com

▶ **Brain Shield Gastrodin**
Life Extension: www.lifeextension.com

▶ **Buffered Vitamin C**
Lypo-Spheric Vitamin C
LivOn Labs: www.livonlabs.com

▶ **Butyri Plex**
American BIologics: www.americanbiologics.com

▶ **Carotenoids**
Betatene
Swanson Health Products: www.swansonvitamins.com

▶ **Collagen**
Collagen JS
Pure Encapsulations: www.pureencapsulations.com

▶ **Colostrum LD**
Sovereign Laboratories: www.sovereignlaboratories.com

▶ **Colostrum Spray**
IRM-Immune Response Modulator
Sovereign Laboratories: www.sovereignlaboratories.com

▶ **Cranberry Extract**
Standardized Cranberry
NOW Foods: www.nowfoods.com

▶ **Cranberry Juice Concentrate**
FruitFast Cranberry Juice Concentrate
Brownwood Acres Foods: www.brownwoodacres.com

▶ **Cresceo-ALC**
Acetyl-L-Carnitine with Vinpocetine
Medix Select: www.medixselect.com

▶ **Curcumin**
CurcumaSorb
Pure Encapsulations: www.pureencapsulations.com

▶ **Derma e Vitamin E Intensive Therapy Body Lotion**
Derma e: www.dermae.com

▶ **DGL Plus**
Pure Encapsulations: www.pureencapsulations.com

▶ **DHA from Fish Oil**
Keralex
Medix Select: www.medixselect.com

▶ **Digestive Enzymes Ultra**
Pure Encapsulations: www.pureencapsulations.com

▶ **DIM-Pro 100**
Pure Encapsulations: www.pureencapsulations.com

▶ **Diosmin and Hesperidin**
DiosVein
Swanson Health Products: www.swansonvitamins.com

▶ **DiosVein**
Swanson Health Products: www.swansonvitamins.comm

▶ **Dr. Ohhira's Probiotic Kampuku Beauty Bar**
Dr. Ohhira Probiotics: www.drohhiraprobiotics.com

▶ **EGCG (Green Tea Extract)**
Teavigo
Pure Encapsulations: www.pureencapsulations.com

▶ **Enzymes for Better Digestion**
Digestive Enzymes Ultra
Pure Encapsulations: www.pureencapsulations.com

▶ **Enzymes for Pain**
Wobenzym N
Wobenzym: www.wobenzym.com

▶ **Eye Formula**
Zeaxanthin Synergistic Eye Formula
Swanson Health Products: www.swansonvitamins.com

▶ **Fish Oil (high DHA)**
Keralex
Medix Select: www.medixselect.com

▶ **Fish Oil (high DHA)**
Super DHA Gems, or
Med Omega Fish Oil
Carlson Nutritional Supplements: www.carlsonlabs.com

▶ **Fish Oil (high EPA)**
Elite EPA Gems
Carlson Nutritional Supplements: www.carlsonlabs.com

▶ **Fish Oil (liquid)**
Carlson's Norwegian Fish Oil, lemon or orange flavored liquid
Carlson Nutritional Supplements: www.carlsonlabs.com

▶ **Fish Oil for Kids**
Carlson for Kids Chewable DHA
Carlson Nutritional Supplements: www.carlsonlabs.com

▶ **Flax Hull Lignans**
Progressive Labs: www.progressivelabs.com

▶ **FruitFast Cranberry Juice Concentrate**
Brownwood Acres Foods: www.brownwoodacres.com

▶ **Garlic**
Kyolic Aged Garlic Extract 100% Vegetarian
Cardiovascular Formula 100
Wakunaga: www.kyolic.com

▶ **Gastrodin**
Brain Shield Gastrodin
Life Extension: www.lifeextension.com

▶ **Ginkgo Biloba**
Ginkgo 50
Pure Encapsulations: www.pureencapsulations.com

▶ **Grape Seed Extract**
Bestvite: www.bestvite.com

▶ **Green Tea Extract**
Teavigo
Pure Encapsulations: www.pureencapsulations.com

▶ **Hairomega DHT**
Hairomega 3-in-1
Bioprosper: www.bioprosper.com

▶ **Heather's Tummy Tamers Peppermint Oil Capsules**
Heather's Tummy Care for IBS: www.heatherstummycare.com

▶ **Hesperidin and Diosmin**
DiosVein
Swanson Health Products: www.swansonvitamins.com

▶ **Imperial Elixir Korean Red Ginseng**
Ginco International: www.gincointernational.com

▶ **IRM Immune Response Modulator**
Sovereign Laboratories: www.sovereignlaboratories.com

▶ **Just Like Sugar®**
Just Like Sugar®: www.justlikesugar.com

▶ **Keralex**
Medix Select: www.medixselect.com

▶ **Korean Red Ginseng**
Imperial Elixir Korean Red Ginseng
Ginco International: www.gincointernational.com

▶ **Kyolic Aged Garlic Extract 100% Vegetarian Cardiovascular Formula 100**
Wakunaga: www.kyolic.com

▶ **Lutein and Zeaxanthin**
Zeaxanthin Synergistic Eye Formula
Swanson Health Products: www.swansonvitamins.com

▶ **Luteolin Complex**
Swanson Health Products: www.swansonvitamins.com

▶ **Lypo-Spheric Vitamin C**
LivOn Labs: www.livonlabs.com

▶ **Magnesium Powder**
Pure Encapsulations: www.pureencapsulations.com

▶ **Magnesium w/SRT**
Jigsaw Health: www.jigsawhealth.com

▶ **Milk Thistle Extract (Silymarin)**
Siliphos
Thorne Research: www.thorne.com

▶ **Multivitamin and Mineral**
Extend Core
Vitamin Research Products: www.vrp.com

▶ **Peppermint Oil Capsules**
Heather's Tummy Tamers
Heather's Tummy Care for IBS: www.heatherstummycare.com

▶ **Probiotic soap**
Dr. Ohhira's Probiotic Kampuku Beauty Bar Soap
Dr. Ohhira Probiotics: www.drohhiraprobiotics.com

▶ **Probiotics**
Theralac
Master Supplements: www.master-supplements.com

▶ **Prostate Revive**
Medix Select: www.medixselect.com

▶ **Pyruvate**
Triple Pyruvate Electrolyte Complex
Swanson Health Products: www.swansonvitamins.com

▶ **Quercetin**
Quercenase
Thorne Research: www.thorne.com

▶ **Redness Relief**
Redness Relief Kit
Zenmed: www.zenmed.com

▶ **Revivogen MD Scalp Therapy**
Revivogen: www.revivogen.com

▶ **Riboflavin 5'-Phosphate (R-5-P)**
Swanson Health Products: www.swansonvitamins.com

▶ **Silver**
Sovereign Silver
Natural Immunogenics: www.natural-immunogenics.com

▶ **Silymarin (Milk Thistle Extract)**
Siliphos
Thorne Research: www.thorne.com

▶ **Soap with Probiotics**
Dr. Ohhira's Probiotic Kampuku Beauty Bar Soap
Dr. Ohhira Probiotics: www.drohhiraprobiotics.com

▶ **Sugar Substitute**
Just Like Sugar®: www.justlikesugar.com

▶ **Sulforaphane**
Swanson Health Products: www.swansonvitamins.com

▶ **Teavigo**
Pure Encapsulations: www.pureencapsulations.com

▸ **Theralac Probiotics**
Master Supplements: www.master-supplements.com

▸ **Triple Pyruvate Electrolyte Complex**
Swanson Health Products: www.swansonvitamins.com

▸ **Vinpocetine with Acetyl-L-Carnitine**
Cresceo-ALC
Medix Select: www.medixselect.com

▸ **Vitamin B2**
Riboflavin 5'-Phosphate (R-5-P)
Swanson Health Products: www.swansonvitamins.com

▸ **Vitamin C**
Lypo-Spheric Vitamin C
LivOn Labs: www.livonlabs.com

▸ **Vitamin E Body Lotion**
Derma e Vitamin E Intensive Therapy Body Lotion
Derma e: www.dermae.com

▸ **Wobenzym N**
Wobenzym: www.wobenzym.com

▸ **Zeaxanthin and Lutein**
Zeaxanthin Synergistic Eye Formula
Swanson Health Products: www.swansonvitamins.com

▸ **Zenmed Redness Relief Kit**
Zenmed: www.zenmed.com

▸ **Zinc Picolinate**
Thorne Research: www.thorne.com

Food Intolerance Testing

Testing can identify delayed, hard-to-connect reactions to foods that are intolerances or sensitivities, rather than immediate allergic reactions. These are some labs that do such testing:

▶ **Alcat**
www.alcat.com

▶ **Genova Diagnostics**
www.gdx.net

▶ **Doctor's Data**
www.doctorsdata.com

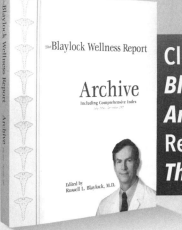
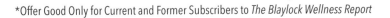